Quality Improvement Research: Understanding the science of change in health care

Edited by

Richard Grol

Professor of Quality in Health Care, Centre for Quality of Care Research (WOK), University Medical Centre St Radboud, Nijmegen; Maastricht University, Maastricht, The Netherlands

Richard Baker

Professor of Quality in Health Care, Department of Health Sciences, University of Leicester, Leicester, UK

Fiona Moss

Associate Dean, North Thames Department of Postgraduate Medical and Dental Education, University of London, London, UK

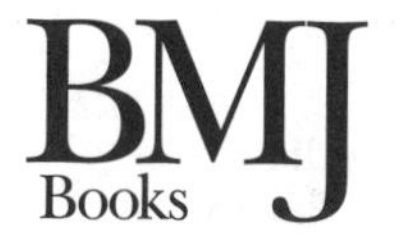

BMJ Books is an imprint of the BMJ Publishing Group

First published in 2004
by BMJ Books, BMA House, Tavistock Square,
London WC1H 9JR

www.bmjbooks.com

British Library Cataloguing in Publication Data

A catalogue record for this book is available from the British Library

ISBN 0 7279 1640 8

Typeset by SIVA Math Setters, Chennai, India
Printed and bound in Spain by GraphyCems, Navarra

Contents

Contributors

Richard Baker
Clinical Governance Research and Development Unit, Department of General Practice and Primary Health Care, University of Leicester, Leicester, UK

James C Benneyan
Quality and Productivity Laboratory, Industrial and Mechanical Engineering, Northeastern University, Boston, Massachusetts, USA

Lisa A Bero
Department of Clinical Pharmacy, University of California, San Francisco, California, USA

Marloes van Bokhoven
Centre for Quality of Care Research (WOK)/Department of General Practice, Maastricht University, Maastricht, The Netherlands

Jozé Braspenning
Centre for Quality of Care Research (WOK), University Medical Centre St Radboud, Nijmegen, The Netherlands

Marion Campbell
Health Services Research Unit, University of Aberdeen, Aberdeen, UK

Stephen Campbell
National Primary Care Research and Development Centre, University of Manchester, Manchester, UK

Huw Davies
Centre for Public Policy and Management, Department of Management, University of St Andrews, Fife, UK

Martin Eccles
Centre for Health Services Research, School of Population and Health Sciences, University of Newcastle upon Tyne, Newcastle upon Tyne, UK

Glyn Elwyn
Department of Primary Care, Swansea Clinical School, Swansea, UK

Roberto Grilli
Department of Clinical Governance, Regional Agency for Health Care of Emilia-Romagna, Bologna, Italy

Jeremy Grimshaw
Clinical Epidemiology Programme, Ottawa Health Research Institute, Ottawa, Canada

Richard Grol
Centre for Quality of Care Research (WOK), University Medical Centre St Radboud, Nijmegen; and Maastricht University, Maastricht, The Netherlands

David Gustafson
Robert Ratner Professor of Industrial Engineering and Preventive Medicine, University of Wisconsin, Madison, USA

Gill Harvey
Manchester Centre for Healthcare Management, University of Manchester, Manchester, UK

Marlies Hulscher
Centre for Quality of Care Research (WOK), University Medical Centre St Radboud, Nijmegen, The Netherlands

Allen Hutchinson
University of Sheffield, Section of Public Health, Sheffield, UK

Gerjo Kok
Department of Experimental Psychology, Maastricht University, Maastricht, The Netherlands

Miranda Laurant
Centre for Quality of Care Research (WOK), University Medical Centre St Radboud Nijmegen, The Netherlands

Robert C Lloyd
Quality Resource Services, Advocate Health Care, Oak Brook, Illinois, USA

Martin Marshall
National Primary Care Research and Development Centre, University of Manchester, Manchester, UK

Laura M McAnley
Institution of population Health, University of Ottawa, Ottawa, Canada

Fiona Moss
North Thames Department of Postgraduate Medical and Dental Education, University of London, London, UK

John Øvretveit
Department of Health Policy and Management, The Nordic School of Public Health, Gothenberg, and The Karolinska Institute, Stockholm, Sweden; and The Faculty of Medicine, Bergen University, Bergen, Norway

Andrew D Oxman
Department of Health Services Research, Directorate for Health and Social Welfare, Oslo, Norway

Paul E Plsek
Paul E Plsek & Associates Inc, Atlanta, Georgia, USA

Catherine Pope
School of Nursing and Midwifery, University of Southampton, Southampton, UK

Alison E Powell
Centre for Public Policy and Management, Department of Management, University of St Andrews, Fife, UK

Craig Ramsay
Health Services Research Unit, University of Aberdeen, Aberdeen, UK

Paul van Royen
Department of General Practice, University of Antwerp, Antwerp, Belgium

Johan L Severens
Department of Health Organisation, Policy and Economics, and Department of Clinial Epidemiology and MTA, University Hospital Maastricht, Maastricht, The Netherlands

Richard Thomson
Department of Epidemiology and Public Health, School of Health Sciences, Medical School, University of Newcastle, Newcastle upon Tyne, UK

Luke Vale
Health Services Research Unit, University of Aberdeen, Aberdeen, UK

Trudy van der Weijden
Centre for Quality of Care Research (WOK)/Department of General Practice, Maastricht University, The Netherlands

Michel Wensing
Centre for Quality of Care Research, University Medical Centre St Radboud, Nijmegen, The Netherlands

Merrick Zwarenstein
Institute for Clinical Evaluative Sciences, Tornoto, Canada

1: Quality improvement research: the science of change in health care

RICHARD GROL, RICHARD BAKER,
FIONA MOSS

We all expect quality these days. "Good enough" care simply is not good enough any more. In consequence, the improvement of patient care has become a major issue in health care in the last decade. Policy reports and articles in leading journals highlight again and again important problems in health care delivery, related to underuse, overuse, and misuse of care.[1]

In fact, the case for quality improvement and change management is broadly accepted by authorities, policy makers, and professionals, and new programmes and policies are constantly being introduced. However, while the management of patients is increasingly expected to be evidence-based, measures and programmes to change practice are more often implemented on the basis of firm beliefs. For instance, for a long time clinical audit with feedback to care providers was the dominant approach to improving quality in many countries, although the benfits from expenditure on this approach have never been adequately evaluated. Programmes aimed at monitoring and improving the quality and safety of patient care are in place in many western countries. They express the different ideas held about, and approaches to, quality improvement that have become popular/fashionable, and include evidence-based medicine, accreditation and (external) accountability, total quality management, professional development and revalidation, risk management and error prevention, organisational development and leadership enhancement, disease management and managed care, complex adaptive systems thinking, or patient empowerment. These approaches differ in perspective. Some focus on changing professionals, others on changing organisations or on changing the interactions between participants in the system. Some emphasise the importance of self regulation in changing care, others believe in the power of external control and incentives. Some prefer bottom-up, others top-down methods for changing practice. But despite their differences, all claim to contribute to better patient care and solve some of its main problems. They may indeed do so, but the evidence for their value, efficiency and feasibility is as yet limited or not studied well.[2] Large sums of money are invested in (educational) programmes and policies without any information about whether the investments are worth the results. On the basis of current evidence none of the approaches to quality improvement can be regarded as superior; we might need all of them to be succesful in achieving quality in health care. However, it is not yet clear which approaches are particularly valid and useful for specific types of changes and for specific target groups and settings.[3]

More evidence and understanding is required to support policy making and implementation of quality improvement policies. We have reasonable knowledge of the effectiveness of selected strategies in the form of more than 50 good systematic reviews and an increasingly large number of controlled trials.[3,4] However, many of the trials can be criticised, for example, because randomisation or analysis were conducted at the patient level, while the intervention focused on professionals or teams. The outcome parameters are often poorly chosen, or difficult to compare. Most studies were performed in the United States, making it difficult to generalise the findings to other healthcare systems. While some strategies have been extensively studied (CME, audit and feedback, reminders and computerised decision support), hardly any good research is available about organisational, economic, administrative and patient-mediated interventions. The effects of new interesting methods such as problem-based education or portfolio learning, TQM approaches, breakthrough projects, risk management methods, business process redesign, organisational development, leadership enhancement, or shared decision making with patients have, so far, not been studied adequately. The current focus on studying the effects of specific strategies in controlled trials provides only part of the answers to our questions about effective change, while they ignore basic questions about critical success factors in change processes.

Health care is becoming more and more complex, so simple improvement measures are seldom effective. The problems related to the improvement of patient care are large. It is therefore not realistic to expect that one specific approach can solve all problems. A qualitative study by Solberg[5] of the critical factors supporting implementation of change showed that a mixture of professional and organisational factors is crucial. "Give attention to many different factors and use multiple strategies", is the message. We have learnt that multifaceted strategies, combining different actions and measures linked to specific obstacles to change, are often successful, but do not have a good understanding of which components of such complex interventions are likely to be effective in different target groups. So, there is some general knowledge about effective change in patient care, but little or no detailed understanding of what is happening within the black box of change. We therefore also need to study change processes in the real world of health care, and learn about the crucial determinants of successful improvement, and about (small) changes related to professionals, patients, social interaction in networks and teams of care providers, and changes related to the systems and structures of health care that can lead to huge improvements in patient care. New thinking about healthcare settings as complex adaptive systems also underline the importance of experimenting with multiple approaches and gradually discovering what is working best.[6] Small changes can sometimes have large effects; we need to find out which small changes, in which settings, can have such impact. In summary, both theories and research findings show that any simple approach to change management is naive and will fail. Well designed interventions need to be developed on the basis of good qualitative work and tested on a small scale before being included in randomised trials or implemented more widely.

That task to be faced requires good research and appropriate, tailored research methodology. Most research on quality improvement has focused, so far, on (audits of) actual care (underuse, overuse, and misuse of care) and determinants of variation in care provision on the one hand, and on studies of the effectiveness of change strategies on the other (mostly trials). Given the complexity of changing practice, it will be clear that additional, less classical research methods and approaches are required. Theoretical models on the evaluation of complex interventions propose a phased approach (theoretical phase, defining components of the intervention, explanatory trial, RCT, long term implementation), with different research methods being used in each phase.[7]

A variety of research methods can be used in quality improvement research:

- observational studies of existing change processes
- in-depth qualitative studies on critical success factors and barriers to change in improvement programmes
- systematic reviews of both the impact of different strategies and the influence of specific factors on change
- well designed cluster randomised trials
- systematic sampling and interpreting experiences with change
- methods for developing valid and sensitive indicators for measuring change
- meta-analyses of large samples of improvement projects
- methods for the evaluation of large scale implementation and change programmes
- economic analyses of the resources needed for effective change and improvement of care.

Research on quality improvement and change management in health care can be regarded as an important new field of health services research, for which the optimal methodology has yet to be established. The expertise of different disciplines, such as epidemiology, social sciences, educational sciences, organisational and management sciences, and economics, is urgently needed. Specific well funded, long term research programmes that stimulate collaboration among researchers in different institutes and in different countries are required to make progress in this very complex field. Reluctance on the part of both research and political organisations to set up and maintain such programmes can, however, be observed in most countries.

To support the thinking and debate about methodologies for quality improvement research, *BMJ* and *Quality and Safety in Health Care* (QSHC) started a joint series of articles on this issue. The series aimed to provide an overview of methodologies that can help us to better understand effective improvement and change in patient care. This book includes the papers published as part of the series.

The science of change management in health care may have passed its infancy, but there is a long way to go before it will provide the crucial answers on how to transform good enough care into high quality care for all patients. We hope that this book will provide help in setting up research to arrive at those answers.

References

1 Bodenheimer T. The American health care system. The movement for improved quality in health care. *N Engl J Med* 1999;**340**:488–92.
2 Grol R. Improving the quality of medical care. Building bridges among professional price, payer profit, and patient satisfaction. *JAMA* 2001; **286**(20):2578–85.
3 Grol R, Grimshaw JM. From best evidence to best practice; about effective implementation of change in patient care. *Lancet* 2003; in press.
4 Grimshaw JM, Shirran L, Thomas R, *et al.* Changing provider behavior: an overview of systematic reviews of interventions. *Med Care* 2001; **39**(suppl 2):II2–45.
5 Solberg L, Brekke M, Fasio J, *et al.* Lessons from experienced guideline implementers: attend to many factors and use multiple strategies. *Jt Comm J Qual Improv* 2000;**26**:171–88.
6 Plsek PE, Greenhalgh T. Complexity science: The challenge of complexity in health care. *BMJ* 2001;**323**:625–8.
7 Campbell M, Fitzpatrick R, Haines A, *et al.* Framework for design and evaluation of complex interventions to improve health. *BMJ* 2000;**321**: 694–6.

2: Research methods used in developing and applying quality indicators in primary care

STEPHEN CAMPBELL, JOZÉ BRASPENNING, ALLEN HUTCHINSON, MARTIN MARSHALL

Quality indicators have been developed throughout Europe primarily for use in hospitals, but also increasingly for primary care. Both development and application are important but there has been less research on the application of indicators. Three issues are important when developing or applying indicators: (1) which stakeholder perspective(s) are the indicators intended to reflect; (2) what aspects of health care are being measured; and (3) what evidence is available? The information required to develop quality indicators can be derived using systematic or non-systematic methods. Non-systematic methods such as case studies play an important role but they do not tap in to available evidence. Systematic methods can be based directly on scientific evidence by combining available evidence with expert opinion, or they can be based on clinical guidelines. While it may never be possible to produce an error free measure of quality, measures should adhere, as far as possible, to some fundamental a priori characteristics (acceptability, feasibility, reliability, sensitivity to change, and validity). Adherence to these characteristics will help maximise the effectiveness of quality indicators in quality improvement strategies. It is also necessary to consider what the results of applying indicators tell us about quality of care.

Quality improvement has become a central tenet of health care. It is no longer the preserve of enthusiastic volunteers but part of the daily routine of all those involved in delivering health care, and has become a statutory obligation in many countries. There are numerous reasons why it is important to improve quality of health care, including enhancing the accountability of health practitioners and managers, resource efficiency, identifying and minimising medical errors while maximising the use of effective care and improving outcomes, and aligning care to what users/patients want in addition to what they need.

Quality can be improved without measuring it – for example, by specialist higher educational programmes such as the vocational training scheme for general practice in the UK or guiding care prospectively in the consultation through clinical guidelines.[1,2] Moreover, there are ways of assessing quality without using hard quantitative measures such as quality indicators – for example, peer review, videoing consultations, patient interviews. Measurement, however, plays an important part in improvement[3,4] and helps to promote change.[5] Specific measures may, for example, allow good performance to be rewarded in a fair way and facilitate accountability. For this reason much effort has gone into developing and applying measures of quality over the last few decades. The purpose of this chapter is to review methods which seek to develop and apply quality indicators.

Defining quality indicators

Indicators are explicitly defined and measurable items which act as building blocks in the assessment of care. They are a statement about the structure, process (interpersonal or clinical), or outcomes of care[6] and are used to generate subsequent review criteria and standards which help to operationalise quality indicators (Box 2.1). Indicators are different from guidelines, review criteria, and standards (Box 2.2). Review criteria retrospectively assess care provided on a case-by-case basis to individuals or populations of patients, indicators relate to care or services provided to patients, and standards refer to the outcome of care specified within these indicators. Standards can be 100% – for example, the National Service Framework for coronary heart disease in the UK has set a standard that all patients with diagnosed coronary heart disease should receive low dose (75 mg) aspirin where clinically appropriate.[7] However, care very rarely meets such absolute standards[8] and, in general, standards should be realistic and set according to local context and patient circumstances.[9,10]

Box 2.1 Definitions of guideline, indicator, review criterion, and standard

Guideline: systematically developed statements to assist practitioner and patient decisions prospectively for specific clinical circumstances; in essence, the "right thing to do".[1,2]

Indicator: a measurable element of practice performance for which there is evidence or consensus that it can be used to assess the quality, and hence change in the quality, of care provided.[9]

Review criterion: systematically developed statement relating to a single act of medical care[9] that is so clearly defined it is possible to say whether the element of care occurred or not retrospectively in order to assess the appropriateness of specific healthcare decisions, services, and outcomes.[110]

Standard: The level of compliance with a criterion or indicator.[9,77,111] A target standard is set prospectively and stipulates a level of care that providers must strive to meet. An achieved standard is measured retrospectively and details whether a care provider met a predetermined standard.

Indicators can measure the frequency with which an event occurred, such as influenza immunisations (activity indicator). However, quality indicators infer a judgement about the quality of care provided.[9] This distinguishes quality indicators from performance indicators,[11] which are statistical devices for monitoring care provided to populations without any necessary inference about quality – for example, they might simply have cost implications. Indicators do not provide definitive answers but indicate potential problems that might need addressing, usually manifested by statistical outliers or perceived unacceptable variation in care. Most indicators have been developed to assess/improve care in hospitals but, increasingly, quality measures are being developed for primary care across Europe.

What should be measured?

There are three important issues to consider when developing indicators. Firstly, which stakeholder perspective(s) are the indicators intended to reflect? There are different stakeholders of health care (patients, carers,

Box 2.2 Examples of a guideline, indicator, review criterion, and standard

Guideline recommendation
If a blood pressure reading is raised on one occasion, the patient should be followed up on two further occasions within x time.

Indicator
Patients with a blood pressure of more than 160/90 mm Hg should have their blood pressure re-measured within 3 months.

Indicator numerator: Patients with a blood pressure of more than 160/90 mm Hg who have had their blood pressure re-measured within 3 months.

Indicator denominator: Patients with a blood pressure of more than 160/90 mm Hg.

Review criterion
If an individual patient's blood pressure was >160/90, was it re-measured within 3 months?

Standard
Target standard: 90% of the patients in a practice with a blood pressure of more than 160/90 mm Hg should have their blood pressure re-measured within 3 months.

Achieved standard: 80% of the patients in a practice with a blood pressure of more than 160/90 mm Hg had their blood pressure re-measured within 3 months.

managers, professionals, third party payers).[3,12] It cannot be presumed that one stakeholder's views represent another group's views.[13,14] Different perspectives may need different methods of indicator development, particularly as stakeholders have different perspectives about quality of care. Health professionals tend to focus on professional standards, health outcomes, and efficiency. Patients often relate quality to an understanding attitude, communication skills, and clinical performance. Managers' views are influenced by data on efficiency, patients' satisfaction, accessibility of care and, increasingly, outcomes. Even if the same aspects of care are assessed, the indicator can be valued differently – for example, health professionals and managers will probably value efficiency differently.

Secondly, which aspects of care should be assessed – processes or outcomes of care?[15–18] The ultimate goal of the care given to patients can be expressed as outcome indicators which measure mortality, morbidity, health status, health related quality of life, and patient satisfaction. Examples include medical outcomes,[19] the outcomes utility index,[20] the Computerized Needs Orientated Quality Measurement Evaluation System,[21] and some of the National Performance Frameworks in the UK.[22] Other outcome indicators include user evaluation surveys derived from systematic literature reviews of patient perspectives of health care[23] or outcome indicators developed using focus groups.[24] In this way items included in validated patient surveys such as the General Practice Assessment Survey[25,26] or Europep[27] can be used as quality indicators. One example of such an indicator might be a patient's capacity to get through to practice staff on the telephone. Structural indicators give information on the practice organisation such as personnel, finances, and availability of appointments.[28–31] For example, if a general practice has a car park there should be specified places for disabled parking. There is limited evidence linking structure with outcomes[32] although research has suggested, for example, a link between longer consultations and higher quality clinical care.[33,34] Process indicators describe actual medical care such as diagnoses, treatment, referral, and prescribing.[10,35] Since our focus is on quality improvement, our main interest in this chapter is on process indicators because improving process has been described as the primary object of quality assessment/improvement.[3,4,16,18,32,36]

Thirdly, in order to develop indicators researchers need information on structure, process, or outcome which can be derived in a number of ways using systematic or non-systematic methods. This information is vital to establish the face or content validity of quality measures (Box 2.3).

Research methods for the development of quality indicators

Non-systematic

Non-systematic approaches to developing quality indicators do not tap in to the evidence base of an aspect of health care; they are based on the availability of data and real life critical

Box 2.3 Definitions of acceptability, feasibility, reliability, sensitivity to change, and validity

Development of quality indicators

- Face/content validity: is the indicator underpinned by evidence (content validity) and/or consensus (face validity)? The extent to which indicators accurately represent the concept being assessed (e.g. quality of care for epilepsy).
- Reproducibility: would the same indicators be developed if the same method of development was repeated?

Application of quality indicators

- Acceptability: is the indicator acceptable to both those being assessed and those undertaking the assessment?
- Feasibility: are valid, reliable, and consistent data available and collectable, albeit contained within medical records, health authority datasets or on videotaped consultations?
- Reliability: minimal measurement error – organisations or practitioners compared with similar organisations or practitioners (comparability), reproducible findings when administered by different raters (inter-rater reliability).
- Sensitivity to change: does the indicator have the capacity to detect changes in quality of care?
- Predictive validity: does the indicator have the capacity for predicting quality of care outcomes?

incidents. This does not mean that they have no useful role in quality assessment/improvement. Examples include quality improvement projects based on one case study.[37] For example, an abortion of a pregnant 13 year old led to a team meeting.[38] Her medical record showed two moments when contraceptives could have been discussed. The response was a special clinic hour for teenagers and the development of a quality indicator on the administration of lifestyle and risk factors. Other examples include many of the high level indicators used by health authorities[39] and referral rates by general practitioners to specialist services in the UK, as well as many of the VIP indicators of practice development in the Netherlands.[29]

Systematic: evidence-based

Where possible, indicators should be based directly upon scientific evidence such as rigorously conducted (trial based) empirical studies.[40–43] The better the evidence, the stronger the benefits of applying the indicators in terms of reduced morbidity and mortality or improved quality of care. For example, patients with confirmed coronary artery disease should be prescribed aspirin, unless contraindicated, as there is evidence that aspirin is associated with improved health benefits in patients with coronary heart disease, although the evidence on the exact dose is unclear. McColl and colleagues have developed sets of evidence-based indicators for use by primary care organisations in the UK based on available data.[44]

Systematic: evidence combined with consensus

There are, however, many grey areas of health care for which the scientific evidence base is limited,[45] especially within the generalist and holistic environment of general practice. This necessitates using an extended family of evidence to develop quality indicators, including utilising expert opinion.[42,46,47] However, experts often disagree on the interpretation of evidence and rigorous and reproducible methods are needed to assess the level of agreement; in particular, combining expert opinion with available evidence using consensus techniques to assess aspects of care for which evidence alone is insufficient, absent, or methodologically weak.[9,41,48] The idea of harvesting professional opinion regarding professional norms of practice to develop quality measures is not new.[3]

Box 2.4 shows that there are a variety of reasons for developing quality indicators using consensus methods. They also allow a wider proportion of aspects of quality of care to be assessed and thus improved than if indicators were based solely on evidence. Quality indicators abound for preventive care, are patchy for chronic care, and are almost absent for acute care in general practice.[49]

Consensus techniques are group facilitation techniques which explore the level of consensus among a group of experts by synthesising and clarifying expert opinion in order to derive a consensus opinion from a group with individual opinions combined into a refined aggregated opinion. Group judgements of professional opinion are preferable to individual practitioner judgements because they are more consistent; individual judgements are more prone to personal bias and lack of reproducibility. Recent examples include

Box 2.4 What are consensus methods designed to do?

- Enhance decision making,[52] develop policies, and estimate unknown parameters.
- Facilitate the development of quality indicators or review criteria[35,61] where evidence alone is insufficient.
- Synthesise accumulated expert opinion/professional norms.[3]
- Identify, quantify, and subsequently measure areas where there is uncertainty,[47] controversy,[53] or incomplete evidence.[112]

quality indicators for common conditions,[10] research on the necessity of process indicators for quality improvement,[50] and a practice visit tool to augment quality improvement.[29]

There are a number of techniques including the Delphi technique[51–53] and the RAND appropriateness method[54] which have been discussed elsewhere,[41] and guideline driven indicators using an iterated consensus rating procedure.[55] The nominal group technique[56] is also used in which a group of experts is asked to generate and prioritise ideas but it is not itself a consensus technique.[41] However, the nominal group technique, supported by postal Delphi, has been used to produce, for example, a national clinical practice guideline in the UK[57] and prescribing indicators.[58]

Delphi technique

The Delphi technique is a structured interactive method involving repetitive administration of anonymous questionnaires, usually across two or three postal rounds. Face to face meetings are not usually a feature. The main stages include identifying a research problem, developing questionnaire statements to rate, selecting appropriate panellists, conducting anonymous iterative postal questionnaire rounds, feeding back results (statistical, qualitative, or both) between rounds, and summarising and feeding back the findings.

The approach enables a large group to be consulted from a geographically dispersed population. For example, Shield and colleagues[59] used 11 panels composed of patients, carers, health managers, and health professionals to rate quality indicators of primary mental health care. Optimal size has not been established and research has been published based on samples ranging from 4 to 3000.

The Delphi procedure permits the evaluation of large numbers of scenarios in a short time period.[60] The avoidance of face to face interaction between group members can prevent individuals feeling intimidated and opinions can be expressed away from peer group pressure. However, the process of providing group and, particularly, individual feedback can be very resource intensive. Moreover, the absence of any face to face panel discussion prohibits the opportunity to debate potentially different viewpoints. There is limited evidence of the validity of quality measures derived using the Delphi technique.[41,52] The Delphi procedure has been used to develop prescribing indicators,[61] managerial indicators,[62] indicators of patient and general practitioner perspectives of chronic illness,[23] indicators for cardiovascular disease,[63] and key attributes of a general practice trainer.[64] The Delphi technique has therefore been used to generate indicators for more than just clinical care.

RAND appropriateness method

This method is a formal group judgement process which systematically and quantitatively combines expert opinion and scientific (systematic literature review) evidence by asking panellists to rate, discuss, and then re-rate indicators. It is the only systematic method of combining expert opinion and evidence.[65] It also incorporates a rating of the feasibility of collecting data, a key characteristic in the application of indicators as discussed below. The main stages include selection of the condition(s) to be assessed, a systematic literature review of the available evidence, generation of preliminary indicators to be rated, selection of expert panels, first round postal survey where panellists are asked to read the accompanying evidence and rate the preliminary indicators, a face to face panel meeting where panellists discuss each indicator in turn, analyses of final ratings, and development of recommended indicators/criteria.[48] The method has been the subject of a number of critiques.[48,65–68]

The RAND method has been used most often to develop appropriateness criteria for clinical interventions in the USA[69,70] such as coronary angioplasty or for developing quality indicators for assessing care of vulnerable elderly patients.[71] It has also been used in the UK,[72–74] including in the development of review criteria for angina, asthma and diabetes[35,75] and for 19 common conditions including acute, chronic, and preventive care.[10]

The strengths of the RAND method are that panellists meet so discussions can take place, no indicators are discarded between rounds so no potential information is lost, and, unlike the standard Delphi technique, panellists are sent a copy of the systematic literature review in addition to the catalogue of indicators. This increases the opportunities for panel members to ground their opinions in the scientific evidence. Research has also shown that using a higher cut-off point for determining consensus within a panel (an overall panel median rating of 8 out of 9) enhances the reproducibility (Box 2.3) of the ratings if a different set of panellists rated the indicators.[76] Shekelle and colleagues found that, while agreement between panels was weak, in terms of kappa values they had greater reliability than many widely accepted clinical procedures such as reading of mammograms.[48]

However, the panels inevitably have to be smaller than the Delphi panels for practical reasons, users/patients are rarely involved, the implications of costs are not considered in ratings, and indicators have been limited to clinical care. Moreover, the face to face nature of the discussion can lead to potential intimidation if there are dominant personalities, although all panellists' ratings carry equal weight irrespective of how much/little they contribute to the discussion.

Systematic: guideline driven indicators

Indicators can be based on clinical guidelines.[55,77–79] Such indicators for general practice have been developed and disseminated widely in the NHS in the UK for four important clinical conditions (diabetes, coronary heart disease, asthma, and depression),[80] using methods proposed by AHCPR.[55] Review criteria were derived from at least one clinical guideline which met a set of quality standards, using structured questions and feedback to test the face and content validity – as well as the feasibility – of the criteria with a panel of over 60 general practitioners.

Hadorn and colleagues[81] described how 34 recommendations in a guideline on heart failure were translated into eight review criteria. Because review criteria must be specific enough to assure the reliability and validity of retrospective review, they used two selection criteria to guide whether each recommendation based criterion should be retained in the final selection – importance to quality of care and feasibility of monitoring. They demonstrated some important aspects of criteria development from guidelines, in particular the need to be very detailed and specific in the criterion, even though the guideline recommendation is less specific and deemed adequate.

Review criteria derived directly from a clinical practice guideline are now part of NHS policy in England and Wales through the work of the National Institute for Clinical Excellence (NICE). Each published summary clinical guideline is accompanied by a set of review criteria which are intended to be used by clinical teams, and the results are externally assessed by the Commission for Health Improvement – for example, in relation to type 2 diabetes.[82] These NICE criteria were developed using an iterated consensus rating procedure similar to that used frequently by the Dutch College of General Practitioners – for example, for back pain and the management of stroke treatment in hospitals. The prominent method in the Netherlands is an iterated consensus rating procedure which seeks to develop indicators based on the impact of guideline recommendations on the outcomes of care (Table 2.1).[55,79] Developers reflect critically on the acceptability of developed sets in conjunction with a group of lay professionals. The method has evolved within the last decade. Some initial studies assessed the performance of the general practitioner on, for example, threatened miscarriage, asthma and chronic obstructive pulmonary disease where the indicator development was limited to the first round of the procedure.[83,84] Other studies used larger panels to assess key recommendations.[85–87] More recent projects have completed all five rounds – for example, a study in which quality indicators were selected for all 70 guidelines developed by the Dutch College of General Practitioners[55] or a study on the management of stroke in hospital.[79,9]

Table 2.1 Guideline driven indicators developed using an iterated consensus rating procedure

	Aim	Undertaken by	Criteria used
Round 1: Pre-selection	Selecting key recommendations	Small group of quality indicators developers (1–3 persons)	Outcome of care: • Patients' health (morbidity, mortality, health status) • Cost
Round 2: Rating and adding	Rating and adding key recommendations	Expert panel (8–10 persons)	• Patients' health • Cost • Sensitivity to change • Availability of data
Round 3: Reliability	Determining inter- and intra-rater reliability	Expert panel for the rating Research team for the analyses	• Kappa, rho
Round 4: Potential indicators	Getting set of potential indicators	Research team	• Cut-off score: mean above mid of rating scale • Agreement among 80% of the panel members
Round 5: Reflection	Acceptability of indicators	Research team Lay professionals	• Face validity

Factors influencing the development of quality indicators using a consensus technique

Many factors influence ratings in a consensus method,[41] especially group composition as groups composed of different stakeholders rating the same statements produce different ratings.[66,88,89] For example, group members who use, or are familiar with, the procedures being rated are more likely to rate them higher.[69,70,89,90] Moreover, panel members from different disciplines make systematically different judgements and feedback from mixed disciplines may influence ratings. For example, a Delphi composed equally of health physicians and managers found that the physicians who had overall feedback, including that of the managers, rated indicators higher than the physicians who had only physician feedback, whereas managers with combined feedback rated lower than managers with only manager feedback.[88]

Ongoing work has provided qualitative evidence of factors which influence individual panellists' ratings in a consensus technique rating aspects of the quality of primary mental health care in a two round postal Delphi.[59] This research used in-depth qualitative interviews with panellists from patient, managerial, and professional panels to identify factors which had influenced panellists' ratings. It concluded that many factors influenced the ratings of the different stakeholder groups (Box 2.5).

Box 2.5 Factors influencing indicators rated valid in a Delphi technique[41,59]

- Composition of the panel
- Inclusion of patient derived (focus group) indicators
- Inclusion of indicators based on "grey" literature
- Inclusion of multiple stakeholders (e.g. patients, carers, managers, health professionals)
- Characteristics of individual panellists (e.g. political perspective, familiarity with research)
- Rating process (e.g. 9 point scale, feedback used)
- Panellists' experience and expectations of the care provision being rated
- Panellists' perspective of the model of care provision
- Panellists' perspective of their locus of control to influence care

Research methods on the application of indicators

Measures derived using expert panels and guidelines have high face validity and those based on rigorous evidence possess high content validity. However, this should be a minimum prerequisite for any quality measure and subsequent developmental work is required to provide empirical evidence, as far as possible, of acceptability, feasibility, reliability, sensitivity to change, and predictive validity (Box 3.3).[6,68,91,92]

Acceptability

The acceptability of the data collected using a measure will depend upon the extent to which the findings are acceptable to both those being assessed and those undertaking the assessment. For example, the iterated consensus rating procedure consults lay professionals as to the acceptability of indicators (Table 3.1). Campbell and colleagues conducted a quality assessment in 60 general practices in England but only used quality indicators rated acceptable and valid by the nurses and doctors working in the practices.[75]

Feasibility

Information about the quality of services is often driven by data availability rather than by epidemiological and clinical considerations.[93] Quality measurement cannot be achieved without accurate and consistent information systems.[15,94] Current administrative data, at both macro (health authority or "large organisation") and micro (individual medical records) levels, are constrained by inconsistent and often unreliable data.[95–98] Medical records are a poor vehicle for collecting data on preventive care and the recording of symptoms.[99–101]

In addition, aspects of care being assessed by quality indicators must relate to enough patients to make comparing data feasible. For example, a clinical audit of angina care excluded 10 criteria rated necessary by an expert panel to provide quality of care[35] because they related to less than 1% of a sample of over 1000 patients in 60 general practices in England.[75]

Reliability

Indicators should be used to compare organisations/practitioners with similar organisations/practitioners, or confounding factors such as socioeconomic and demographic factors, as well as factors outside the control of practitioners, should be taken into account (that is, compare like with like or risk/case mix adjust). This is because the environment in which an organisation operates affects the care provided. Examples include admission rates or surgery rates. Indicators must also have explicit exclusion and inclusion criteria for applying the indicator to patients – for example, age ranges, co-morbidities, case mix, and clinical diagnoses.

The inter-rater reliability of an indicator can also be tested when applying indicators. For example, in a study of over 1000 patients with diabetes two raters abstracted data separately (but on the same day) for 7·5% of all patient records and found that five criteria out of 31 developed using an expert panel were excluded from analyses due to poor agreement.[75]

Sensitivity to change

Quality measures must be capable of detecting changes in quality of care[17] in order to discriminate between and within subjects.[91] This is an important and often forgotten dimension of Lawrence's definition of a quality indicator.[9]

Validity

There has been little methodological scrutiny of the validity of consensus methods.[42,46,92,102] The Delphi technique[103] and the RAND method[16,104] have both been criticised for a lack of evidence of validity. While the issue has received more attention in recent years,[6,16,36] there is little evidence for the validity of the Delphi method in developing quality indicators.

Content validity of indicators generated using consensus techniques

Content validity in this context refers to whether any indicators were rated by panels contrary to known results from randomised controlled trials. There is evidence for the content validity of indicators derived using the RAND method.[48,105]

Predictive validity

There is evidence of the predictive validity of indicators developed using the RAND method.[48,106,107] For example, Kravitz and colleagues studied a cohort of persons who had undergone coronary angiography. Patients were retrospectively classified as to whether coronary revascularisation was "necessary" or "not necessary" according to the review criteria, and outcomes at year 1 were measured. Patients meeting the "necessary" criteria for coronary revascularisation who did not receive it were twice as likely to have died at 1 year as those who did receive "necessary" revascularisation. Hemingway and colleagues[74] found substantial underuse of coronary revascularisation among UK patients who were considered appropriate for these procedures and underuse was associated with adverse clinical outcomes on the basis of the ratings of an expert panel.

Using data generated by applying quality indicators

Data generated using quality indicators can be used for a variety of purposes – for example, to monitor, reward, penalise, or compare care provision (perhaps using league tables or public release of data) or as part of a quality improvement strategy. Simply measuring something will not automatically improve it. Indicators must be used within coherent systems based approaches to quality improvement.[108,109] The interpretation and usage of such data is more of a political or resource issue than a methodological or conceptual one.

The provenance of the indicators is important when applying them. Indicators derived from informal consensus procedures with little evidence underlying them might be useful as educational guidelines. However, the best indicators for public disclosure, for use in league tables, or for attaching financial incentives are those based solely on scientific evidence, for which the implications of applying the indicator and any relative judgements that are be inferred about the results can be confidently predicted. Indicators derived from consensus methods which systematically combine evidence and opinion may also be disclosed, but perhaps with more provisos. Indicators developed by well respected experts using a systematic method might also have high credibility when used for professional development.

Conclusion

It may never be possible to produce an error free measure of quality, but measures should adhere, as far as possible, to some fundamental a priori characteristics in their development (face/content validity) and application (acceptability, feasibility, reliability, sensitivity to change, predictive validity). Adherence to these characteristics will help maximise the effectiveness of quality indicators in quality improvement strategies. This is most likely to be achieved when they are derived from rigorous scientific evidence. However, evidence in health care is often absent. We believe that using consensus techniques – which systematically combine evidence and opinion – and guideline driven approaches facilitates quality improvement. They allow a significantly broader range of aspects of care to be assessed and improved than would be the case if quality indicators were restricted to scientific evidence.

It is important that such methods of development continuously improve and seek to incorporate advances in the evidence base of health care. However, it may be that research has reached a peak in developing indicators. There is much less research on the application of indicators and their reliability, validity, and effectiveness in quality improvement strategies, how indicators can be used to improve care, and how professionals/service users can be helped to be more engaged with the development and use of indicators. Introducing strategies for quality improvement based on quality indicators does not make them effective and successful without understanding the factors that are required to underpin their development and to facilitate their transference between settings and countries.

Key messages

- Most quality indicators have been developed in hospitals but they are increasingly being developed for primary care in Europe and the USA.
- Most research has focused on the development rather than the application of indicators.
- Quality indicators should be based on rigorous scientific evidence if possible. However, evidence in health care is often absent, necessitating the use of other methods of development including consensus techniques (such as the Delphi technique and the RAND appropriateness method) which combine expert opinion and available evidence and indicators based on clinical guidelines.
- While it may never be possible to produce an error free measure of quality, measures should adhere, as far as possible, to some fundamental a priori characteristics – namely, acceptability, feasibility, reliability, sensitivity to change, and validity.
- The way in which indicators are applied is as important as the method of development.

References

1 Forrest D, Hoskins A, Hussey. Clinical guidelines and their implementation. *Postgrad Med J* 1996;**72**:19–22.
2 Grimshaw JM, Russell IT. Effect of clinical guidelines on medical practice: a systematic review of rigorous evaluations. *Lancet* 1993;**342**:1317–22.
3 Donabedian A. *Explorations in quality assessment and monitoring*. Volume 1: The definition of quality and approaches to its assessment. Ann Arbor, Michigan: Health Administration Press, 1980.
4 Irvine D. *Managing for quality in general practice*. London: King's Fund Centre, 1990.
5 Juran JM. *Juran on planning for quality*. New York: Free Press, 1988.
6 McGlynn EA, Asch SM. Developing a clinical performance measure. *Am J Prevent Med* 1998;**14**:14–21.
7 Department of Health. *A National Service Framework for coronary heart disease*. London: Department of Health, 2000.
8 Seddon ME, Marshall MN, Campbell SM, *et al*. Systematic review of studies of clinical care in general practice in the United Kingdom, Australia and New Zealand. *Qual Health Care* 2001;**10**:152–8.
9 Lawrence M, Olesen F, *et al*. Indicators of quality health care. *Eur J Gen Pract* 1997;**3**:103–8.
10 Marshall M, Campbell SM. Introduction to quality assessment in general practice. In: Marshall M, Campbell SM, Hacker J, Roland MO, eds. *Quality indicators for general practice: a practical guide for health professionals and managers*. London: Royal Society of Medicine, 2002:1–6.
11 Buck D, Godfrey C, Morgan A. *Performance indicators and health promotion targets*. Discussion paper 150. York: Centre for Health Economics, University of York, 1996.

12 Øvretveit J. *Health service quality: an introduction to quality methods for health services*. Oxford: Blackwell Scientific Publications, 1992.
13 McGlynn EA. Six challenges in measuring the quality of health care. *Health Aff* 1997;**16**:7–21.
14 Joss R, Kogan M. *Advancing quality: total quality management in the National Health Service*. Buckingham: Open University Press, 1995.
15 Davies HTO, Crombie IK. Assessing the quality of care. *BMJ* 1995;**311**:766.
16 Eddy DM. Performance measurement: problems and solutions. *Health Aff* 1998;**17**:7–26.
17 Mant J, Hicks N. Detecting differences in quality of care: the sensitivity of measures of process and outcome in treating acute myocardial infarction. *BMJ* 1995;**311**:793–6.
18 Palmer RH. Process-based measures of quality: the need for detailed clinical data in large health care databases. *Ann Intern Med* 1997;**127**:733–8.
19 Tarlov AR, Ware JE, Greenfield S, *et al*. The Medical Outcomes Study: an application of methods for monitoring the results of medical care. *JAMA* 1989;**262**:925–30.
20 McGlynn EA. The outcomes utility index: will outcomes data tell us what we want to know? *Int J Qual Health Care* 1998;**10**:485–90.
21 Agency for Healthcare Research and Quality. *Computerized needs: oriented quality measurement evaluation system*. Rockville: Agency for Healthcare Research and Quality, 1999. http://www.ahrq.gov/qual/conqix.htm
22 NHS Executive. *Quality and performance in the NHS: high level performance indicators*. London: Department of Health, 1999.
23 Roland MO, Holden J, Campbell SM. *Quality assessment for general practice: supporting clinical governance in primary care groups*. Manchester: National Primary Care Research and Development Centre, 1998.
24 Wensing M, Jung HP, Mainz J, *et al*. A systematic review of the literature on patient priorities for general practice care. Part 1: Description of the research domain. *Soc Sci Med* 1998;**47**:1573–88.
25 Campbell SM, Hann M, Hacker J, *et al*. Identifying predictors of high quality care in English general practice: an observational study. *BMJ* 2001;**323**:784–7.
26 Ramsay J, Campbell JL, Schroter S, *et al*. The General Practice Assessment Survey (GPAS): tests of data quality and measurement properties. *Fam Pract* 2000;**17**:372–9.
27 Wensing M, Vedsted P, Kersnik J, *et al*. Patient satisfaction with availability of general practice: an international comparison. *Int J Qual Health Care* 2002;**14**:111–8.
28 National Committee for Quality Assurance. *Narrative: What's in it and why it matters*. Volume 1. HEDIS 3.0/1998. Washington: National Committee for Quality Assurance, 1998.
29 Van den Hombergh P, Grol R, van den Hoogen HJ, *et al*. Practice visits as a tool in quality improvement: mutual visits and feedback by peers compared with visits and feedback by non-physician observers. *Qual Health Care* 1999;**8**:161–6.
30 American Academy of Family Physicians. *The Family Practice Management Practice Self-Test*. 2001 http://www.aafp.org/fpm/20010200/41thef.html
31 Royal Australian College of General Practitioners. *Standards for general practice*. Royal Australian College of General Practitioners, 2000.
32 Brook RH, McGlynn EA, Cleary PD. Measuring quality of care. *N Engl J Med* 1996;**335**:966–70.
33 Howie JG, Heaney DJ, Maxwell M. Measuring quality in general practice. Pilot study of a needs, process and outcome measure. *Occasional Paper of the Royal College of General Practitioners* 1997;**75**:1–32.

34 Wilson A, Childs S. *Systematic review on consultation length in general practice*. A report to the Scientific Foundation Board of the RCGP. Leicester: University of Leicester, 2001.
35 Campbell SM, Roland MO, Shekelle PG, *et al*. Development of review criteria for assessing the quality of management of stable angina, adult asthma and non-insulin dependent diabetes in general practice. *Qual Health Care* 1999;**8**:6–15.
36 Brook RH, McGlynn EA, Shekelle PG. Defining and measuring quality of care: a perspective from US researchers. *Int J Qual Health Care* 2000;**12**: 281–95.
37 Pringle M. Preventing ischaemic heart disease in one general practice: from one patient, through clinical audit, needs assessment, and commissioning into quality improvement. *BMJ* 1998;**317**:1120–4.
38 Pringle M. Clinical governance in primary care. Participating in clinical governance. *BMJ* 2000;**321**:737–40.
39 NHS Executive. *Quality and performance in the NHS: high level performance indicators*. London: Department of Health, 1999.
40 Hearnshaw HM, Harker RM, Cheater FM, *et al*. Expert consensus on the desirable characteristics of review criteria for improvement of health quality. *Qual Health Care* 2001;**10**:173–8.
41 Campbell SM, Cantrill JA. Consensus methods in prescribing research. *J Clin Pharm Ther* 2001;**26**:5–14.
42 Murphy MK, Black NA, Lamping DL, *et al*. Consensus development methods, and their use in clinical guideline development. *Health Technol Assess* 1998;**2**(3).
43 Baker R, Fraser RC. Is ownership more important than the scientific credibility of audit protocols? A survey of medical audit advisory groups. *Fam Pract* 1997;**14**:107–11.
44 McColl A, Roderick P, Gabbay J, *et al*. Performance indicators for primary care groups: an evidence-based approach. *BMJ* 1998;**317**:1354–60.
45 Naylor CD. Grey zones in clinical practice: some limits to evidence based medicine. *Lancet* 1995;**345**:840–2.
46 Black N, Murphy M, Lamping D, *et al*. Consensus development methods: a review of best practice in creating clinical guidelines. *J Health Serv Res Policy* 1999;**4**:236–48.
47 Jones JJ, Hunter D. Consensus methods for medical and health services research. *BMJ* 1995;**311**:376–80.
48 Shekelle PG, Kahan JP, Bernstein SJ, *et al*. The reproducibility of a method to identify the overuse and underuse of procedures. *N Engl J Med* 1998;**338**:1888–95.
49 Campbell SM, Roland MO, Buetow S. Defining quality of care. *Soc Sci Med* 2000;**51**:1611–25.
50 Ibrahim JE. Performance indicators form all perspectives. *Int J Qual Health Care* 2001;**13**:431–2.
51 Linstone HA, Turoff M. *The Delphi survey. Method, techniques and applications*. Reading, Massachusetts: Addison-Wesley, 1975.
52 Hasson F, Keeney S, McKenna H. Research guidelines for the Delphi survey technique. *J Adv Nurs* 2000;**32**:1008–15.
53 Fink A, Kosecoff J, Chassin M, *et al*. Consensus methods: characteristics and guidelines for use. *Am J Public Health* 1984;**74**:979–83.
54 Brook RH, Chassin MR, Fink A, *et al*. A method for the detailed assessment of the appropriateness of medical technologies. *Int J Technol Assess Health Care* 1986;**2**:53–63.
55 Braspenning J, Drijver R, Schiere AM. *Quality indicators for general practice* (in Dutch). Nijmegen/Utrecht: Centre for Quality of Care Research/ Dutch College of General Practitioners, 2001.

56 Delbecq AL, Van de Ven AH, Gustafson D. *Group techniques for programme planning: a guide to nominal group and Delphi processes*. Glenview, Illinois: Scott, Foresman & Company, 1975.
57 Department of Health. *Treatment choice in the psychological therapies and counselling*. London: Department of Health, 2001.
58 Cantrill JA, Sibbald B, Buetow S. Indicators of the appropriateness of long term prescribing in general practice in the United Kingdom: consensus development, face and content validity, feasibility and reliability. *Qual Health Care* 1998;**7**:130–5.
59 Shield T, Campbell SM, Rogers A, Gask L. Quality indicators for mental health care in primary care. *Qual Saf Health Care*, 2003;**12**:100–6.
60 Rockwell MA. The Delphi procedure: knowledge from goat viscera? *N Engl J Med* 1973;**288**:1298–9.
61 Campbell SM, Cantrill JA, Richards D. Prescribing indicators for UK general practice: Delphi consultation study. *BMJ* 2000;**321**:1–5.
62 Campbell SM, Roland MO, Quayle JA, *et al*. Quality indicators for general practice. Which ones can general practitioners and health authority managers agree are important and how useful are they? *J Public Health Med* 1998;**20**:414–21.
63 Normand SL, McNeil BJ, Peterson LE, *et al*. Eliciting expert opinion using the Delphi technique: identifying performance indicators for cardiovascular disease. *Int J Qual Health Care* 1998;**10**:247–60.
64 Munro N, Hornung RI, McAteer S. What are the key attributes of a good general practice trainer? A Delphi study. *Educ Gen Pract* 1998;**9**: 263–70.
65 Naylor CD. What is appropriate care? *N Engl J Med* 1998;**338**:1918–20.
66 Hicks NR. Some observations on attempts to measure appropriateness of care. *BMJ* 1994;**309**:730–3.
67 Ayanian JZ, Landrum MB, Normand SLT, *et al*. Rating the appropriateness of coronary angiography – do practicing physicians agree with an expert panel and with each other? *N Engl J Med* 1998;**338**:1896–904.
68 Campbell SM. *Defining, measuring and assessing quality of care in general practice*. PhD Thesis, University of Manchester, 2002.
69 Leape LL, Hilborne LH, Schwartz JS, *et al*. The appropriateness of coronary artery bypass graft surgery in academic medical centres. *Ann Intern Med* 1996;**125**:8–18.
70 Kahn KL, Rogers WH, Rubenstein LV, *et al*. Measuring quality of care with explicit process criteria before and after implementation of a DRG-based prospective payment system. *JAMA* 1990;**264**:1969–73.
71 Shekelle PG, MacLean CH, Morton SC, *et al*. Assessing care of vulnerable elders: methods for developing quality indicators. *Ann Intern Med* 2001;**135**:647–52.
72 Gray D, Hampton JR, Bernstein SJ, *et al*. Audit of coronary angiography and bypass surgery. *Lancet* 1990;**335**:1317–20.
73 Scott EA, Black N. Appropriateness of cholecystectomy in the United Kingdom: a consensus panel approach. *Gut* 1991;**32**:1066–70.
74 Hemingway H, Crook AM, Feder G, *et al*. Underuse of coronary revascularization procedures in patients considered appropriate candidates for revascularization. *N Engl J Med* 2001;**344**:645–54.
75 Campbell SM, Hann M, Hacker J, *et al*. Quality assessment for three common conditions in primary care: validity and reliability of review criteria developed by expert panels for angina, asthma and type 2 diabetes. *Qual Saf Health Care* 2002;**11**:125–30.
76 Shekelle PG, Kahan JP, Park RE, *et al*. Assessing appropriateness by expert panels: how reliable? *J Gen Intern Med* 1996;**10**:81.

77 Eccles M, Clapp Z, Grimshaw J, *et al*. North of England evidence based guidelines development project: methods of guideline development. *BMJ* 1996;**312**:760–2.
78 Agency for Healthcare Research and Quality. *Using clinical practice guidelines to evaluate quality of care*. Volume 2: Methods. Rockville: Agency for Healthcare Research and Quality, 1995.
79 CBO Quality Institute for Health Care. *Handbook. Development of indicators on evidence-based guidelines* (in Dutch). Utrecht: Quality Institute for Health Care, 2002.
80 Hutchinson A, Anderson JP, McIntosh A, *et al*. *Evidence based review criteria for coronary heart disease*. Sheffield: Royal College of General Practitioners Effective Clinical Practice Unit, University of Sheffield, 2000.
81 Hadorn DC, Baker DW, Kamberg CJ, *et al*. Phase II of the AHCPR-sponsored heart failure guideline: translating practice recommendations into review criteria. *Jt Comm J Qual Improv* 1996;**22**:265–76.
82 National Institute for Clinical Excellence. *Management of type 2 diabetes: renal disease-prevention and early management*. London: National Institute for Clinical Excellence, 2002.
83 Smeele IJ, Grol RP, van Schayck CP, *et al*. Can small group education and peer review improve care for patients with asthma/chronic obstructive pulmonary disease? *Qual Health Care* 1999;**8**:92–8.
84 Grol R, Dalhuijsen J, Thomas S, *et al*. Attributes of clinical guidelines that influence use of guidelines in genral practice: observational study. *BMJ* 1998;**317**:858–61.
85 Spies TH, Mokkink HGA. *Using guidelines in clinical practice* (in Dutch). Nijmegen/Utrecht: Centre for Quality of Care Research/Dutch College of General Practitioners, 1999.
86 Schers H, Braspenning J, Drijver R, *et al*. Low back pain in general practice: reported manegement and reasons for not adhering to the guidelines in the Netherlands. *Br J Gen Pract* 2000;**50**:640–4.
87 Frijling BD, Spies TH, Lobo CM, *et al*. Blood pressure control in treated hypertensive patients: clinical performance of general practitioners. *Br J Gen Pract* 2001;**51**:9–14.
88 Campbell SM, Hann M, Roland MO, *et al*. The effect of panel membership and feedback on ratings in a two-round Delphi survey. *Med Care* 1999;**37**:964–8.
89 Coulter I, Adams A, Shekelle P. Impact of varying panel membership on ratings of appropriateness in consensus panels: a composition of a multi- and single disciplinary panel. *Health Serv Res* 1995;**30**:577–91.
90 Fraser GM, Pilpel D, Kosecoff J, *et al*. Effect of panel composition on appropriateness ratings. *Int J Qual Health Care* 1994;**6**:251–5.
91 Streiner DL, Norman GR. *Health measurement scales: a practical guide to their development and use*. Oxford: Oxford Medical Publications, 1995.
92 Huff ED. Comprehensive reliability assessment and comparison of quality indicators and their components. *J Clin Epidemiol* 1997;**50**:1395–404.
93 Siu AL, McGlynn EA, Morgenstern H, *et al*. Choosing quality of care measures based on the expected impact of improved care on health. *Health Serv Res* 1992;**27**:619–50.
94 Thomson R, Lally J. Clinical indicators: do we know what we're doing? *Qual Health Care* 1998;**7**:122.
95 Enthoven AC. A promising start, but fundamental reform is needed. *BMJ* 2000;**320**:1329–21.
96 Wilkinson EK, McColl A, Exworthy M, *et al*. Reactions to the use of evidence-based performance indicators in primary care: a qualitative study. *Qual Health Care* 2000;**9**:166–74.

97 Baker R. Managing quality in primary health care: the need for valid information about performance. *Qual Health Care* 2000;**9**:83.
98 Craddock J, Young A, Sullivan G. The accuracy of medical record documentation in schizophrenia. *J Behav Health Serv Res* 2001;**28**: 456–66.
99 Wyatt JC, Wright P. Design should help use of patients' data. *Lancet* 1998;**352**:1375–8.
100 Wu L, Ashton CM. Chart review: a need for reappraisal. *Evaluating Health Professionals* 1997;**20**:146–63.
101 Luck J, Peabody JW, Dresselhaus TR, *et al.* How well does chart abstraction measure quality? A prospective comparison of standardized patients with the medical record. *Am J Med* 2000;**108**:642–9.
102 Salzer MS, Nixon CT, Schut LJA, *et al.* Validating quality indicators: quality as relationship between structure, process and outcome. *Evaluation Rev* 1997;**21**:292–309.
103 Kahn KL, Park RE, Vennes J, *et al.* Assigning appropriateness ratings for diagnostic upper gastrointestinal endoscopy using two different approaches. *Med Care* 1992;**30**:1016–28.
104 Phelps CE. The methodologic foundations of studies of the appropriateness of medical care. *N Engl J Med* 1993;**329**:1241–5.
105 Merrick NJ, Fink A, Park RE, *et al.* Derivation of clinical indications for carotid endarterectomy by an expert panel. *Am J Public Health* 1987; **77**:187–90.
106 Kravitz RL, Laouri M, Kahan JP, *et al.* Validity of criteria used for detecting underuse of coronary revascularization. *JAMA* 1995;**274**: 632–8.
107 Selby JV, Fireman BH, Lundstrom. Variation among hospitals in coronary-angiography practices and outcomes after myocardial infarction in a large health maintenance organisation. *N Engl J Med* 1996;**335**:1888–96.
108 Ferlie EB, Shortell SM. Improving the quality of health care in the United Kingdom and the United States: a framework for change. *Milbank Quarterly* 2001;**79**:281–315.
109 Campbell SM, Sweeney GM. The role of clinical governance as a strategy for quality improvement in primary care. *Br J Gen Pract* 2002; **52**(suppl):S12–S17.
110 Donabedian A. *Explorations in quality assessment and monitoring*. Volume 2: The criteria and standards of quality. Ann Arbor, Michigan: Health Administration Press, 1982.
111 Donabedian A. The quality of medical care. *Science* 1978;**200**:856–64.
112 Lomas J, Anderson G, Enkin M, *et al.* The role of evidence in the consensus process. Results from a Canadian consensus exercise. *JAMA* 1988;**259**:3001–5.

3: Using routine comparative data to assess the quality of health care: understanding and avoiding common pitfalls

ALISON POWELL, HUW DAVIES, RICHARD THOMSON

Measuring the quality of health care has become a major concern for funders and providers of health services in recent decades as a result of a number of diverse and interrelated developments. These include the increasing range of treatment options, growing pressure on resources, and the introduction of new structures for delivering and monitoring health care. One of the ways in which quality of care is currently assessed is by taking routinely collected data and analysing them quantitatively. The use of routine data has many advantages but there are also some important pitfalls. Collating numerical data in this way means that comparisons can be made – whether over time, with benchmarks, or with other healthcare providers (at individual or institutional levels of aggregation). Inevitably, such comparisons reveal variations. The natural inclination is then to assume that such variations imply rankings: that the measures reflect quality and that variations in the measures reflect variations in quality. This paper identifies reasons why these assumptions need to be applied with care, and illustrates the pitfalls with examples from recent empirical work. It is intended to guide not only those who wish to interpret comparative quality data, but also those who wish to develop systems for such analyses themselves.

The pressures facing healthcare funders and providers are mounting. Not only is health care itself becoming more complex, with an increasing range of new treatment options and competing approaches to the delivery of care, but care must also be delivered in a context of cost constraints, increasing consumer demands, and a greater focus on accountability. Against this background there has been an explosion in official and unofficial schemes aiming to use routine data to compare performance between healthcare providers.[1,2] Such data can help highlight any problem areas in clinical performance, inform or drive quality improvement activities, prompt reflections on clinical practice, and identify important issues for further research. These data thus have a wide range of potential uses and are of interest to a wide range of stakeholders – researchers, practitioners, managers, purchasers, policy makers, patients, and carers.

The logic underlying an analysis of routine comparative data is that it is possible to make attributions of causality between the services provided and the observed quality measures – that is, that high *measured* performance reflects good *actual* performance – and, conversely, that low measured performance reflects poor actual performance. For example, if one hospital has markedly better survival rates 30 days after myocardial infarction than another, then one conclusion from the data might be that the higher survival rates result from higher quality care at the first hospital. But how well founded is this conclusion? What are the difficulties that arise in developing schemes that can draw robust conclusions from routinely collected comparative data? This paper will consider a range of potential pitfalls. Using examples from recent studies of quality variations we explore the risks and benefits of using routine comparative data to draw conclusions about quality of health care.

Using routine data in health services

The use of routine data for quality assessment purposes is attractive to researchers, health professionals, managers, and policy makers. Box 3.1 summarises the reasons: the data are readily available, they are a potentially rich source of information about large numbers of patients, and using existing data is less demanding (and has fewer ethical constraints) than planning, funding, and executing long term experimental studies.

Box 3.1 Reasons for use of routine data for quality assessment purposes

- The data are readily available in many healthcare settings (although accuracy and completeness may vary).
- They can be used retrospectively whereas experimental designs by definition have to be set up prospectively; thus data for large time periods can be gathered more quickly than in a new study.
- Because the data are in many cases already being collected for other purposes, the costs of setting up data collection and retrieval systems are likely to be much lower.
- The data are a rich source of information about large numbers of patients with different conditions across diverse geographical and healthcare settings.
- Ethical and consent issues applying to routine data are less problematic than those which apply to data gathering primarily for research purposes.

What routine data have in common is that they are often collected for other purposes and are observational rather than experimental. Examples of routine data collected in the UK NHS, to take just one healthcare system, include perioperative deaths, hospital bed occupancy rates, use of contraceptive services in general practice, cervical screening, and vaccination rates (see, for example, the latest government collated data at http://www.doh.gov.uk/performanceratings/2003/index.html). In the USA, routine data collection includes state specific initiatives – for example, the California Hospital Outcomes Project reports public data on a range of indicators including 30 day mortality after myocardial infarction[3,4] – and national programmes – for example, the national register for myocardial infarction supported by Genentech.[5] In addition, the Joint Commission on Accreditation of Healthcare Organizations (JCAHO) requires hospitals to submit clinical performance data on six measures,[6] and extensive measures are collected to help compare health plans.[7] Indicators derived from routine data may cover processes of care (for example, treatments given, length of hospital stay), "true" outcomes (for example, mortality rates), or "proxy" outcomes (for example, physiological measures such as blood pressure or weight gain). In quality assessment terms process measures – which assess, for example, what was done and when (how quickly or how often) – may be most illuminating if there is definite evidence for providing a particular drug treatment or intervention.[8] Outcome measures may be more useful if there is a clear temporal and causal link between the care given and the outcome achieved, and if there is consensus about the value to the patient and/or the service of the outcome studied.[9] In any case, routine data impose certain interpretation limitations on both process and outcome measures, although these limitations may operate in different ways.[10]

Issues in interpreting routine data to assess quality of care

Whether attempting to gain understanding from published comparisons of performance or designing new schemes to analyse routine data to allow such comparisons, we need to understand how the ways in which data are collected may impact on the interpretations that are possible. A clear understanding of the potential pitfalls arising may allow some of these to be anticipated and avoided during system design, or can temper the conclusions drawn from established schemes. Four main issues affect the interpretation of comparative routine data:

- measurement properties
- controlling for case mix and other relevant factors
- coping with chance variability
- data quality.

Measurement properties

The development and validation of indicators is dealt with in Chapter 2. Two key measurement concerns apply when routine data are used for quality purposes: (1) the validity and reliability of the outcome measures themselves; and (2) the risk of conflicting findings when different measures are used to assess the same organisations.

Validity and reliability

Routine data provide a given set of variables from which quality measures can be selected or derived. Yet poor validity and/or reliability of the measures can undermine the conclusions drawn. Common threats to validity and reliability may arise from many sources – for example, from the fact that such data are usually collected unblinded. When outcome assessors are aware of previous treatment histories there is empirical evidence that this may affect the judgements reached.[11] Furthermore, when providers are aware that they will be judged on the data, other incentives may come into play leading to concerns about "gaming" with data.[12]

Inappropriate data sources may add to measurement concerns, either overestimating or underestimating services provided. Hospital discharge forms, for example, which are produced for billing and other administrative purposes, may lack the important clinical details needed for quality assessment.[13,14] In one study of medical and surgical hospital discharges, a tool commonly used in the USA to analyse computerised hospital discharge abstracts (the Complications Screening Program) failed to pick up instances of substandard care that were evident when the same patients' medical records were reviewed according to explicit criteria.[15] Another study in primary care which set out to determine the optimal method of measuring the delivery of outpatient services found that medical records had low sensitivity for measuring health counselling but moderate sensitivity for some other aspects including laboratory testing and immunisation.[16] In contrast, self-completed patient exit questionnaires had mixed sensitivity for laboratory testing but moderate to high sensitivity for health counselling and immunisation.

Even apparently "hard" and valid end points like death can be problematic. A study of routine data on in-hospital deaths[17] found that this measure gave an incomplete reflection of mortality within 30 days of admission for surgery, and that the measure was less valid in more recent years than historically. "In-hospital deaths" are usually defined as deaths in the admission in which surgery was performed, but counting only these deaths excludes those that occur elsewhere – whether at home or in other hospitals after transfer – but which may nonetheless be related to the operative care. Since these statistics were first collected in the 1960s and 1970s, shorter hospital stays and an increased tendency to transfer patients between hospitals for specialist care mean that a greater proportion of deaths within 30 days of admission for surgery will be missed if the original definition is used.

Additional problems arise because some clinical conditions, particularly chronic problems, may require a range of interventions provided by different health professionals, both in hospital and in the community, and thus may not be amenable to a single quality measure. For example, the US Health Plan Employer Data and Information Set (HEDIS), which is used across a range of services, was found to have low validity as a tool by which to assess behavioural healthcare quality after hospital admission for major affective disorder.[18]

The validity of quality measures derived from routine data may be further undermined by changes in reporting practices over time. In a study of emergency admissions in one health authority from 1989/90 to 1997/8 an apparent increase in emergency activity was not matched by an increase in the number of admissions or by the increase in the number of patients each year.[19] What appeared to be a rise in emergency admissions turned out to be mainly due to increased reporting of internal transfers after admission.

The validity of routine data may also be compromised by differences in data gathering practice between providers. A study of nosocomial (hospital acquired) infection[20] suggests that it is difficult to make meaningful comparisons between hospitals in relation to reported infection rates as the infection surveillance practices vary so much. The study investigated whether there was a relationship between surveillance practices and reported nosocomial infection rates but concluded that any such relationship was not systematic: "there appears to be a serious issue regarding the equivalency of the data collection processes".[20]

The overriding message from these examples is the need to establish beforehand the validity, reliability, sensitivity, and other metric properties of any proposed measures. Wherever possible, indicators drawn from routine data should be tested against freshly gathered data using "gold standard" measures with well established metric properties.

Conflicting findings

Routine data sets may provide a wide variety of potential measures on which to assess quality of care – for example, quality of surgical services may be assessed using early or longer term mortality, duration of ICU stay, complications, or infection rates. Yet studies using routine data suggest that there may be little correlation between different outcomes, with the effect that the same institution may look good on some indicators and poor on others[21] – for example, there may be little or no correlation between hospital mortality rates and complication rates.[22] This means that the ranking of institutions and the selection of those requiring further quality review may largely depend on the specific measures chosen for review. When data are being used for exploration and insight, such conflicting messages may simply offer a rich source of avenues for further investigation. However, if the intention is to seek to make definitive judgements on performance, then the potential for conflicting findings suggests the need to make decisions on primary end points at the design stage (much as is now commonplace in the design of prospective randomised controlled trials).

Controlling for case mix and other relevant factors

Even when concerns over validity and reliability have been satisfied, there is a further threat to the meaningful interpretation of routine data. Performance comparisons between healthcare providers need to take into account whether the measures being compared derive from similar patient groups: clinical and other characteristics of the patients treated are likely to affect both the demands placed on the service and, in particular, the outcomes from treatment. In observational studies these case mix differences cannot be controlled for at the outset as they are through randomisation in prospective trials, so retrospective risk adjustment is required instead. Such systems usually rely on developing some kind of scoring system that encapsulates the level of risk the patient faces, irrespective of any care delivered. Clearly, accounting for these factors, which are outside the control of those providing the care, is essential before any comparison of the outcome of care is possible.

Various patient characteristics have been recognised as important in increasing risk, such as age, disease severity, co-morbidities, and past medical history. Scoring systems are designed to quantify a number of discrete but interrelated patient characteristics and reduce these to a single value reflecting the overall severity of the condition or risk that the patient faces. For each scoring system the association between the independent variables (patient characteristics) and the dependent variable (the outcome of interest, often death) is described in the form of a mathematical model known as a multiple logistic regression model. The mathematical model describes the strength of the association of each of the different independent variables with the dependent variable, while allowing for the effect of all the other independent variables in the same model. The weights or coefficients associated with the independent variables in the model are derived from analysis of large databases of past patients containing information on both the patient factors required for the scoring system and the outcomes of interest. These models must then be calibrated before being assessed for their sensitivity and specificity – most usefully, this testing procedure should be carried out on new cohorts of patients. Needless to say, developing and testing such scoring schemes is highly technical and complex, and requires substantial statistical expertise. Developing robust schemes thus introduces a wide range of challenges which are reviewed in detail elsewhere.[13,22]

Sophisticated risk adjustment models take a long time to create, test, and implement. It is necessary to know which aspects of case mix have any bearing on outcomes in order to know whether to adjust for these in any given patient group and to what extent, either singly or in combination with other factors. Further, the usefulness of the risk adjustment model is only as good as the underlying assumptions on which it is based, which means that there has to be a priori knowledge that a particular factor is relevant. For many diagnoses the necessary information is not yet available to create robust risk adjustment models.

Even with a reasonably robust risk adjustment model, the data demands of risk adjustment pose their own challenges which may increase as the complexity of the model increases. Sophisticated risk adjustment requires detailed information about which patients had these characteristics in the first place. This information is rarely routinely available – either because at the time the data were collected this particular characteristic was not thought to be relevant, or because the data set is incomplete or inaccurate in certain aspects. The concerns over validity and reliability of measures explored earlier apply as much, if not more, to the variables collected for risk adjustment as they do to the outcome measures themselves.

A further difficulty arises when different risk adjustment schemes lead to different rankings of performance. To take one example, risk adjusted mortality rates may not be a good measure of hospital quality of care as severity can be defined in quite different ways and different severity adjustment schemes may lead to different judgements.[22] This is well illustrated in a study which showed that the same patients were assigned markedly differing risks of dying after coronary artery bypass graft surgery, acute myocardial infarction, pneumonia, and stroke, depending on the severity measure used.[23] This resulted in conflicting impressions of relative hospital performance.

While such concerns are not always seen empirically – for example, other studies have found that hospital rankings remained stable irrespective of the severity measure used[24,25] – it is difficult to be confident about which severity adjustment scheme is the most valid. In any case, even when risk adjustment is carried out, the risk remains of confounding from significant unknown (and therefore unadjusted) factors. In a complex field like health care, the predictive power of even the best risk adjustment models will only ever be partial.

Risk adjustment is not only a complex problem in itself, but it is also a dynamic problem. The process of using risk adjusted figures to make comparisons over time is hampered by the problem of "upstaging" – that is, the grading of patients over time may shift upwards, perhaps because of greater attention being given to the initial assessment of severity. As the definitions of severity drift upwards, the highest risk patients in one category are moved up to the next highest risk category where they are lower risk relative to the other patients in the group. The highest risk patients from that group get moved up too, so each risk category loses some of its most severe cases and gains less severe cases. The outcomes (for example, mortality and morbidity) for each risk category considered separately thus appear to improve as the "pool" of severity within them is diluted. Such severity difference or "upstaging" has been seen in relation to coronary artery bypass graft surgery in New York State where some of the apparent improvements in mortality were in part attributed to drifts in severity assessments.[26] Guarding against upstaging in any given study may require periodic checking of the validity and reliability of any assessment tools to check for any drifts in grading practice.

Despite the considerable challenges involved in clinically credible risk adjustment, ignoring the issue is not an option: inadequate case mix adjustment can have a significant effect on the conclusions drawn from routine data. A review of seven published observational studies reporting a reduced mortality with increased volume of coronary artery bypass graft surgery found that the apparent benefit of receiving treatment in high volume hospitals decreased as the degree of case mix adjustment increased.[27] Furthermore, the size of the estimated benefit of treatment in a high volume centre reduced over time. Concluding that the estimates of benefit suggested in the literature are likely to be misleading because of inadequate adjustment for case mix, these authors and others[28,29] warn that other observational studies using routine data may overestimate the effect of high volumes of activity on the quality of health care.

Non-clinical factors can also have a major impact on quality measures, both in conjunction with case mix issues and independently of them. Yet adjusting for many of these factors can be harder than adjusting for clinical factors, leaving the possibility that apparently poorly performing hospitals may be penalised for factors outside their control. For example, in the USA community sociodemographic factors which impacted on patient physical and mental health status were found to have more influence on admission rates than physician practice styles.[30] Studies of admission rates to hospitals from different general practices in London show that much of the variation in hospital admission rates between GP practices is explicable by differences in patient populations, with a higher prevalence of chronic illness and deprivation being associated with higher admission rates.[31,32]

Added to these patient-specific characteristics which may affect quality assessments are confounding contextual factors over which health providers may have little or no control, such as the availability of services within that facility and in adjacent health or social care services. A study of the extent to which measures of population health, demographic characteristics, socioeconomic factors, and secondary care characteristics influenced admission rates from general practice[33] found that these factors explained substantial proportions of the variations between health authorities in admission rates for epilepsy, asthma, and diabetes (55%, 45%, and 33%, respectively). A further example exploring variations in cervical smear uptake rates among general practices found that there was marked variation between practices with rates ranging from 17% to 94%. Yet, using a multiple regression model, over half of this variation could be accounted for by patient and practice variables – notably the presence or absence of a female partner within the practice.[34]

In addition to adjusting for case mix, there is also therefore a need to think through broader system and contextual influences and how these may alter, diminish, or otherwise undermine the conclusions that can be drawn about variations. The outcome of such deliberations may lead to collection of a wider data set of potential confounders to allow exploration of some of these wider influences.

Coping with chance variability

Chance variability is present in all data and can hinder interpretation of routine data in two ways: (1) by showing apparent differences that are not real and (2) by obscuring real differences.

False alerts

Ranking or other comparisons arising from routine data contain de facto tests of hypotheses of difference. Yet statistical theory shows that when two units – for example, institutions or services – are compared, statistically significant differences will be seen one time in 20 (assuming the usual significance levels of 0·05 are used), even when there is no true difference between them. Routine data are therefore prone to identifying false outliers which may lead to hospitals being inappropriately praised or denigrated (the statistical "type I error"). This problem is obviously compounded when multiple comparisons are made, which is common in studies of healthcare quality. For example, in one study of acute myocardial infarction, Monte Carlo simulation modelling found that over 75% of hospitals assessed as "poor quality" on the strength of their high mortality rates for this condition were actually of average quality.[35] In a separate study evaluating the predictive power of early readmission rates in cardiac disease, around two thirds of hospitals labelled poor quality due to their outlier status on this measure were also found to be falsely labelled.[36] Even when providers are statistically worse than average, the extent of divergence not attributable to chance may be quite small. For example, death rates following congestive heart failure or acute myocardial infarction were 5–11% higher in one set of hospitals than in all other hospitals and yet, for each of these, most of the excess (56–82%) was compatible with purely random variation.[37]

The potentially misleading effects of multiple testing (leading to frequent type I errors) can largely be avoided by pre-specifying the key outcomes of interest and testing statistical significance only for these. Comparisons beyond this limited set are then treated more as hypothesis *raising* than as hypothesis *testing*.

False reassurance

In addition to producing false outliers, chance can also hide real and important differences in quality within random fluctuations. Routine data are prone to providing false reassurance where important differences are not detected (statistically, the "type II error"). Thus, conventional statistical tests may fail to detect instances where hospital care is poor – for example, a hospital which fails to provide treatments which are known to be effective – because they concentrate on outcomes and these may appear within statistical norms when taken across disparate units. One study which used an analytical model to explore the sensitivity and predictive power of mortality rate indicators[38] found that fewer than

12% of poor quality hospitals emerged as high mortality rate outliers (indicating a high rate of type II errors), while over 60% of the "poor" outliers were in fact good quality hospitals (another high rate of type I errors).

For statistical reasons, differences in reported rates may or may not be statistically significant depending on how many years' data are used.[22,33] Depending on what is being assessed, large patient numbers (and hence long time periods) may be required to be able to detect a difference. This may be inappropriate at the institutional level (as staff and facilities change) and impractical at the individual physician level. For example, in relation to a chronic disease like diabetes, it may be difficult to develop a reliable measure to assess physician performance and routine data may show little evidence either way.[39]

A priori power calculations can help determine how much data will be needed to say something meaningful about differences.[40] Such calculations made at the design stage can ensure that sufficient data can be collected to uncover potentially important differences. A crucial part of such a power calculation is the specification of what magnitude of difference would be regarded as *clinically* (as opposed to merely *statistically*) significant.

That outcome measures can be highly data demanding was well illustrated in a paper by Mant and Hicks[41] which used the management of acute myocardial infarction as an example to compare the relative sensitivity of measures of process and outcome in detecting deficiencies in care. The authors concluded that "even with data aggregated over three years, with a perfect system of severity adjustment and identical case ascertainment and definition, disease specific mortality is an insensitive tool with which to compare quality of care among hospitals".[41] The lesson that arises from such an observation is that systems designers should choose variables for which there is most likely to be a high degree of variability – which should lead to earlier emergence of any significant differences.

Real change or statistical artefact?

Comparisons of quality are not just about snapshots of practice; they are also intended to convey the extent of any changes in performance over time. Yet the problem of disentangling real change from statistical artefact is demonstrated in a study of the estimated adjusted live birth rate for 52 in vitro fertilisation clinics, the subsequent clinic ranking, and the associated uncertainty.[42] The researchers found that the confidence intervals were wide, particularly for those clinics placed in the middle ranks, and hence there was a high degree of uncertainty associated with the rankings. For example, one unit which fell in the middle of the rankings (27/52) had a 95% confidence interval for its rank ranging from 16 to 37. Furthermore, assessing changes in ranking in successive years also proved difficult. Looked at over two successive years, with only two exceptions, "changes (in clinic ranking) of up to 23 places (out of the 52) were not associated with a significant improvement or decline in adjusted live birth rate".[42]

Finally, the statistical phenomenon of "regression to the mean" will also account for some of the apparent movement of services up or down the rankings over a period of years[43] – so again not all observed changes are prima facie evidence of quality improvement or deterioration. While there are technical approaches that can, to some extent, adjust for such a phenomenon,[44,45] they are not simple and suggest the need for early statistical support at the design stage.

Data quality

The interpretation of comparative routine data thus faces three major challenges: (1) the need for appropriate measures; (2) the need to control for case mix and other variables, and (3) the need to minimise chance variability. These are all underpinned by a fourth challenge – namely, the need for high quality data. It is self-evident that poor quality data compound the inherent problems of interpretation of routine data described above and can undermine even the most sophisticated quality assessment tool. Yet, even in well resourced, well organised research studies, it is difficult to ensure that data are complete and of a consistently high quality.[9] It is harder still to ensure that routine data are of a high standard; the many factors that can compromise the reliability of both primary and secondary data have been well described.[22] For example, those collecting and entering the data are likely to be doing so as one of many daily tasks; data collection may be in conflict with other priorities and limited understanding of the purpose of the data may lead to unwitting errors in non-standard situations. Many different individuals will be involved in data collection and recording over long time periods and the risks of mistakes and inconsistencies or gaps are high. Thus, when routine data are used for quality assessment purposes, it is a common finding that they are inaccurate, with omissions and erroneous inclusions, or incomplete (especially in relation to some treatments) or insufficiently detailed for the purpose.[46]

Recent studies suggest that these difficulties persist. One study looked at whether the clinical conditions represented by the coding on hospital discharge summaries were actually present, as confirmed by clinical evidence in medical records. It found that, of 485 randomly sampled admissions, although there was clinical evidence to support most coded diagnoses of postoperative acute myocardial infarction, confirmatory evidence was lacking in at least 40% of other diagnoses, calling into question the interpretation of quality measures based on those diagnoses.[47]

Another recent study that looked at the accuracy of tumour registry data found that tumour registries provided largely accurate data on hospital based surgical treatment but there were large gaps in the data for outpatient treatments.[48] For example, the overall rate of radiation therapy after breast conserving surgery was found to be 80% when fresh data were gathered but was originally reported for only 48% of cases in the registry data. For adjuvant therapy the figures also diverged with less than one third of those who had in fact received adjuvant therapy having this information recorded within the registries. Tumour registries thus had significant omissions, particularly in failing to reflect adequately the care provided in outpatient settings.

Despite the importance of achieving accuracy in data collection, many studies have highlighted the fact that processes for routine data collection are still developing. One recent study which looked at 65 community health "report cards" in the USA[49] found that there were significant variations across all areas, with data collection being the biggest challenge, and only half of the communities used pre-existing formats or the experience of others to guide report card development. The authors concluded that improved infrastructure and greater systematisation of the process would make it more sustainable. As these challenges appear to be significant in many settings, an early assessment of data quality is an essential first step for those seeking to exploit routine data sources for comparative studies of quality.

Concluding remarks

Comparative data on the quality of health care serve many purposes and have the potential to both provide insight and drive quality improvement activities. Nonetheless, we have described a range of reasons why such judgements should be made with care. Deficiencies in measurement properties, problems with case mix, the clouding effects of chance, and the sometimes precarious nature of the underlying data sources all raise issues of concern (summarised in Box 3.2).

Given the many problems surrounding the interpretation of routine data to assess healthcare quality, does this point towards the use of process measures or outcome measures? It is clear that concerns about data quality apply to both. Beyond this, it is the interpretation of outcome measures which is most susceptible to the serious threats posed by issues of validity and reliability, the confounding effects of case mix and other factors, and the problem of chance variability. For example, although process measures require the definition of appropriate processes of care for specific patient groups, the problem of case mix largely ends there. Adjusting for case mix in outcomes studies can be far more complex. Furthermore, whereas assessments of processes going awry can often be made from relatively small numbers, assessing such failures from outcomes alone requires much larger studies.[10,41] Process measures are also relatively easy to interpret, and they provide a direct link to the remedial action required. They may be particularly useful in revealing quality problems that are not susceptible to outcome measurement – for example, "near misses", unwanted outcomes, or unnecessary resource use.[10]

Another distinct problem with outcome measurement in terms of quality improvement and performance management

Box 3.2 Variations in measured quality: real difference or artefact?

When routine data reveal variations between different service providers in reported quality measures, this may be evidence of real differences in quality of care. Other possible causes of variation include:

(1) Problems with measurement: validity and reliability of measures can be undermined by:

- inappropriate/insensitive data sources, e.g. data taken from administrative systems may lack necessary clinical details;
- measures which are too narrow to reflect the care provided, e.g. using a single measure in psychiatric care;
- inappropriate/insensitive definition of outcomes, e.g. looking at 30 day mortality for a particular condition even when most deaths fall outside this period;
- changes in data recording over time, e.g. apparent improvement or deterioration because of changes in reporting practices;
- differences in data recording between providers, e.g. data collection processes may not be equivalent and may lead to apparent variations;
- lack of blinding, e.g. unblinded assessment of outcome is prone to bias.

(2) The presence of case mix and other factors: apparent differences between units may be more attributable to differences in the patient groups – for example, in clinical and sociodemographic terms and in terms of contextual factors – than to any true differences in performance. Yet case mix adjustment is demanding:

- it is always incomplete as adjustment can only be made when the necessary data are available and when the relevant factors are known;
- the choice of adjustment scheme can itself affect quality rankings;
- all adjustment schemes risk "upstaging" where the severity grading of patients may drift upwards over time, with implications for severity adjusted outcomes.

(3) Chance variability: this can lead to falsely identifying outliers for praise or blame (type I errors) or can obscure real differences and thus hide poor performers (type II errors).

(4) Poor data quality: despite growing awareness of the problem, routine data systems are often incomplete or inaccurate, and this can seriously undermine conclusions drawn from such data.

is that, in many cases, the outcomes of interest are much delayed. While early postoperative mortality may be close to the point of intervention, many other key outcome measures are far removed from the period of clinical care. Re-operations for recurrent inguinal hernia or second joint replacement procedures, for example, usually occur late after surgery. Another pertinent example would be the use of survival to monitor the outcomes of cancer therapies, often measured several years after treatment. This is not to deny that these are important measures of outcome for patients and health systems. However, the fundamental problem in terms of performance management or quality improvement is that, by the time these measures are available, they will reflect clinical practice of several years previously and hence have extremely limited capacity to influence the clinical practice that led to them. Thus, if quality assessment in health care is to mature, the enthusiasm for outcomes data will need to be tempered by due recognition of the complementary benefits of process data.

Clearly, many of the potential pitfalls highlighted in this paper can be overcome through (1) the development of indices with better metric properties, (2) more sophisticated risk adjustment, and (3) gathering more data and using alternative forms of statistical assessment such as control charts.[50–52] The success of each of these in turn rests upon high quality, locally derived and used, detailed clinical data sets.[46] Identifying the potential pitfalls, as we have done, highlights where most attention must be paid for quality researchers to ensure that the comparisons produced are robust and reliable indicators of real variations in quality practice.

Crucially, this paper has been concerned simply with the *interpretation* of apparent quality variations. We have not addressed the utility or utilisation of such comparative analyses, their proper role in local or national quality improvement efforts, or the scope for public involvement in their interpretation. Each of these issues is complex and contested.[53–56] Yet debates surrounding the use of such comparative analyses could be facilitated by a clearer understanding of the information content of routine data. It is to this end that the analysis presented is addressed.

Key messages

- Observational data assessing healthcare quality often show wide variations between geographical regions, healthcare providers, and even individual practitioners.
- Some of these variations may reflect real and important variations in actual healthcare quality, variations that merit further investigation and action.
- Apparent variation may also arise because of other misleading factors such as variations in sampling, differences in the validity and reliability of measures, or unadjusted case mix differences.
- Measures of process may be less susceptible to spurious variations than measures of outcome.
- Separating real from artefactual variations can be tricky, and judgements about the quality of care should therefore always be made with caution when using routine comparative data.

Potential conflict of interest: Richard Thomson is the Director of the UK Quality Indicator Project, a branch of the International Quality Indicator Project, which provides anonymised feedback of comparative indicator data to UK hospitals.

References

1 Davies HT, Marshall MN. Public disclosure of performance data: does the public get what the public wants? *Lancet* 1999;**353**:1639–40.
2 Nutley SM, Smith PC. League tables for performance improvement in health care. *J Health Serv Res Policy* 1998;**3**:50–7.
3 Rainwater JA, Romano PS, Antonius DM. The California Hospital Outcomes Project: how useful is California's report card for quality improvement? *Jt Comm J Qual Improve* 1998;**24**:31–9.
4 Romano PS, Rainwater JA, Antonius D. Grading the graders: how hospitals in California and New York perceive and interpret their report cards. *Med Care* 1999;**37**:295–305.
5 Davies HT. Public release of performance data and quality improvement: internal responses to external data by US health care providers. *Qual Health Care* 2001;**10**:104–10.
6 Kohn LT, Corrigan JM, Donaldson MS, eds. *To err is human: building a safer health system*. Washington, DC: National Academy Press, 2000.
7 NCQA. *HEDIS. The health plan employer data and information set*. Washington, DC: National Committee for Quality Assurance, 1999.
8 Davies HT, Crombie IK. Assessing the quality of care. *BMJ* 1995;**311**:766.
9 Davies HT, Crombie IK. Interpreting health outcomes. *J Eval Clin Pract* 1997;**3**:187–99.
10 Crombie IK, Davies HT. Beyond health outcomes: the advantages of measuring process. *J Eval Clin Pract* 1998;**4**:31–8.

11 Noseworthy J, Ebers G, Vandervoort M, *et al.* The impact of blinding on the results of a randomized, placebo-controlled multiple sclerosis clinical trial. *Neurology* 1994;**44**:16–20.
12 Smith P. On the unintended consequences of publishing performance data in the public sector. *Int J Public Admin* 1995;**18**:277–310.
13 Leyland AH, Boddy FA. League tables and acute myocardial infarction. *Lancet* 1998;**351**:555–8.
14 Jenkins KJ, Newburger JW, Lock JE, *et al.* In-hospital mortality for surgical repair of congenital heart defects: preliminary observations of variation by hospital caseload. *Pediatrics* 1995;**95**:323–30.
15 Iezzoni LI, Davis RB, Palmer RH, *et al.* Does the complications screening program flag cases with process of care problems? Using explicit criteria to judge processes. *Int J Qual Health Care* 1999;**11**:107–18.
16 Stange KC, Zyzanski SJ, Fedirko Smith T, *et al.* How valid are medical records and patient questionnaires for physician profiling and health services research? A comparison with direct observation of patient visits. *Med Care* 1998;**36**:851–67.
17 Goldacre MJ, Griffith M, Gill L, *et al.* In-hospital deaths as fraction of all deaths within 30 days of hospital admission for surgery: analysis of routine statistics. *BMJ* 2002;**324**:1069–70.
18 Druss B, Rosenheck R. Evaluation of the HEDIS measure of behavioural care quality. *Psychiatr Serv* 1997;**48**:71–5.
19 Morgan K, Prothero D, Frankel S. The rise in emergency admissions – crisis or artefact? Temporal analysis of health services data. *BMJ* 1999;**319**:158–9.
20 Wakefield DS, Hendryx MS, Uden-Holman T, *et al.* Comparing providers' performance: problems in making the "report card" analogy fit. *J Healthcare Qual* 1996;**18**:4–10.
21 Hartz AJ, Kuhn EM. Comparing hospitals that perform coronary artery bypass surgery: the effect of outcome measures and data sources. *Am J Publ Health* 1994;**84**:1609–14.
22 Iezzoni LI. Using risk-adjusted outcomes to assess clinical practice: an overview of issues pertaining to risk adjustment. *Ann Thorac Surg* 1994;**58**:1822–6.
23 Iezzoni LI. The risks of risk adjustment. *JAMA* 1997;**278**:1600–7.
24 Shwartz M, Iezzoni LI, Ash AS, *et al.* Do severity measures explain differences in length of hospital stay? The case of hip fracture. *Health Services Res* 1996;**31**:365–85.
25 Iezzoni LI, Shwartz M, Ash AS, *et al.* Does severity explain differences in hospital length of stay for pneumonia patients? *J Health Serv Res Policy* 1996;**1**:65–76.
26 Green J, Wintfeld N. Report cards on cardiac surgeons: assessing New York State's approach. *N Engl J Med* 1995;**332**:1229–32.
27 Sowden AJ, Deeks JJ, Sheldon TA. Volume and outcome in coronary artery bypass graft surgery: true association or artefact? *BMJ* 1995;**311**:151–5.
28 Posnett J. Is bigger better? Concentration in the provision of secondary care. *BMJ* 1999;**319**:1063–5.
29 Spiegelhalter DJ. Mortality and volume of cases in paediatric cardiac surgery: retrospective study based on routinely collected data. *BMJ* 2002;**324**:261–4.
30 Komaromy M, Lurie N, Osmond D, *et al.* Physician practice style and rates of hospitalization for chronic medical conditions. *Med Care* 1996;**34**:594–609.
31 Reid FDA, Cook DG, Majeed A. Explaining variation in hospital admission rates between general practices: cross sectional study. *BMJ* 1999;**319**:98–103.

32 Majeed A, Bardsley M, Morgan D, *et al.* Cross sectional study of primary care groups in London: association of measures of socioeconomic and health status with hospital admission rates. *BMJ* 2000;**321**:1057–60.
33 Giuffrida A, Gravelle H, Roland M. Measuring quality of care with routine data: avoiding confusion between performance indicators and health outcomes. *BMJ* 1999;**319**:94–8.
34 Majeed F, Cook D, Anderson H, *et al.* Using patient and general practice characteristics to explain variations in cervical smear uptake rates. *BMJ* 1994;**308**:1272–6.
35 Hofer TP, Hayward RA. Identifying poor-quality hospitals: can hospital mortality rates detect quality problems for medical diagnoses? *Med Care* 1996;**34**:737–53.
36 Hofer TP, Hayward RA. Can early re-admission rates accurately detect poor-quality hospitals? *Med Care* 1995;**33**:234–45.
37 Park RE, Brook RH, Kosecoff J, *et al.* Explaining variations in hospital death rates. Randomness, severity of illness, quality of care. *JAMA* 1990;**264**:484–90.
38 Thomas JW, Hofer TP. Accuracy of risk-adjusted mortality rate as a measure of hospital quality of care. *Med Care* 1999;**37**:83–92.
39 Hofer TP, Hayward RA, Greenfield S, *et al.* The unreliability of individual physician 'report cards' for assessing the costs and quality of care of a chronic disease. *JAMA* 1999;**281**:2098–105.
40 Florey CdV. Sample size for beginners. *BMJ* 1993;**306**:1181–4.
41 Mant J, Hicks N. Detecting differences in quality of care: the sensitivity of measures of process and outcome in treating acute myocardial infarction. *BMJ* 1995;**311**:793–6.
42 Marshall EC, Spiegelhalter DJ. Reliability of league tables of in vitro fertilisation clinics: retrospective analysis of live birth rates. *BMJ* 1998;**316**:1701–5.
43 Bland JM, Altman DG. Statistics notes: Regression towards the mean. *BMJ* 1994;**308**:1499.
44 Bland JM, Altman DG. Statistics notes: Some examples of regression towards the mean. *BMJ* 1994;**309**:780.
45 Hayes RJ. Methods for assessing whether change depends on initial value. *Stat Med* 1988;**7**:915–27.
46 Black N. High-quality clinical databases: breaking down barriers. *Lancet* 1999;**353**:1205–6.
47 McCarthy EP, Iezzoni LI, Davis RB, *et al.* Does clinical evidence support ICD-9-CM diagnosis coding of complications? *Med Care* 2000;**38**:868–87.
48 Bickell NA, Chassin MR. Determining the quality of breast cancer care: do tumor registries measure up? *Ann Intern Med* 2000;**132**:705–10.
49 Fielding JE, Sutherland CE, Halforn N. Community health report cards: results of a national survey. *Am J Prev Med* 1999;**17**:79–86.
50 Mohammed MA, Cheng KK, Rouse A, *et al.* Bristol, Shipman, and clinical governance: Shewhart's forgotten lessons. *Lancet* 2001;**357**:463.
51 Adab P, Rouse AM, Mohammed MA, *et al.* Performance league tables: the NHS deserves better. *BMJ* 2002;**324**:95–8.
52 Lawrance RA, Dorsch MF, Sapsford RJ, *et al.* Use of cumulative mortality data in patients with acute myocardial infarction for early detection of variation in clinical practice: observational study. *BMJ* 2001;**323**: 324–7.
53 Mannion R, Davies HTO. Report cards in health care: learning from the past; prospects for the future. *J Eval Clin Pract* 2002;**8**:215–28.
54 Davies HTO, Bindman AB, Washington AE. Health care report cards: implications for the underserved and the organizations who provide for them. *J Health Politics Policy Law* 2002;**27**:379–99.

55 Marshall MN, Davies HTO. Public release of information on quality of care: how are the health service and the public expected to respond? *J Health Serv Res Policy* 2001;6:158–62.
56 Lally J, Thomson RG. Is indicator use for quality improvement and performance measurement compatible? In: Davies HTO, Tavakoli M, Malek M, *et al*, eds. *Managing quality: strategic issues in health care management*. Aldershot: Ashgate, 1999:199–214.

4: Qualitative methods in research on healthcare quality

CATHERINE POPE, PAUL VAN ROYEN, RICHARD BAKER

There are no easy solutions to the problem of improving the quality of care. Research has shown how difficult it can be, but has failed to provide reliable and effective ways to change services and professional performance for the better. Much depends on the perspectives of users and the attitudes and behaviours of professionals in the context of their organisations and healthcare teams. Qualitative research offers a variety of methods for identifying what really matters to patients and carers, detecting obstacles to changing performance, and explaining why improvement does or does not occur. The use of such methods in future studies could lead to a better understanding of how to improve quality.

> I went to see Roy Griffiths (architect of the 1984 NHS reforms and supermarket chief executive) in his office at Sainsbury's and while I was talking to him his secretary handed him a piece of paper. He looked at it and said: "OK". I asked him: "What do you mean OK?" and he said: "My organisation is OK today". It turned out he had just six measures on that piece of paper and from those he could tell what the state of Sainsbury's health had been the day before; things like the amount of money taken yesterday, the freshness quotient – the amount of stuff on the shelves – the proportion of staff on duty and so on.
>
> NHS regional manager quoted in Strong and Robinson.[1]

The above quote illustrates a view of management in the retail sector that was seen in the UK in the 1980s as a role model for health services. The quality of health care could be assured if we could only develop good quantitative measures such as performance indicators, and thus identify problems, make changes, and improve health services. This vision has been tempered with the realisation that the issue of "quality" is more complicated and nebulous than this model of management implies, especially in the case of complex health systems and services. The assessment of quality of services can no longer be confined simply to monitoring such aspects as waiting time, but requires an understanding of the experience of waiting for care – for example, the nature of the clinical environment, the adequacy of communication by and with health professionals, the context and manner in which treatment is delivered, and whether services and care meet expectations. Moreover, it is increasingly recognised that views of quality depend on one's perspective: patients, providers, politicians, and the public may all have contested views of what constitutes high or poor quality care.

The concept of quality in health care is multidimensional and complex and some of the questions we want to ask about the quality of care or services may not be amenable to quantitative measurement. Qualitative research has come to the fore in health and social research by providing ways of answering these sorts of questions,[2,3] both in the form of "standalone" or independent research projects and as a complement to quantitative studies.

The use of qualitative methods in qualitative research involves the systematic collection, organisation, and analysis of textual material derived from talk or observation. It is rooted in the interpretive perspectives found in the humanities and social sciences that emphasise the importance of understanding, from the viewpoint of the people involved, how individuals and groups interpret, experience, and make sense of social phenomena. It is not possible here to elaborate on the origins and theoretical underpinnings of this distinctive approach to research, but it is important to be aware that qualitative research is informed by a quite different paradigm to that which governs quantitative clinical and biomedical research. The emphasis in qualitative research on understanding meanings and experiences makes it particularly useful for quality assessment and for unpacking some of the complex issues inherent to quality improvement. This paper explores some of the qualitative methods that can help to gather information about the delivery of good quality health care and explain variations in healthcare provision.

The methods

Qualitative researchers study phenomena and events in their natural settings, often interpreting them in terms of the subjective meanings attached by the individual. Qualitative methods for collecting data include interviews, observation, and analysis of documents. Different methods may be appropriate to different situations and different research questions. In some cases a single method may be used while in others a combination of methods may be employed. In this chapter we focus on interview based and observational methods as these are the most commonly used in quality assessment.

Interview based methods

Individual face to face interviews may be either semi-structured or in-depth. Semi-structured interviews are typically based on a flexible topic guide that provides a loose structure of open ended questions to explore experiences and attitudes. In-depth interviews provide an opportunity to obtain more detail about an issue or experience, and are especially useful for exploring experiences of care. Because this method elicits people's own views and accounts, it can have the additional benefit of uncovering issues or concerns that had not been anticipated or considered by the researchers. In order to ensure that really detailed information is gathered, interview methods require experienced researchers with the necessary sensitivity and ability to establish rapport with respondents, to use topic guides flexibly, and to follow up questions and responses.

Focus groups are similar in structure to face to face interviews but they use the interaction of a group of, typically, 6–8 people to generate data. This allows group members to talk to one another, argue, and ask questions, and is especially useful for finding out about shared experiences. Focus groups have been successfully used with users and staff. One adaptation of this method is the "exploration group" in which different healthcare providers who have direct contact with a particular health problem review and discuss some material such as audio or video taped cases or interviews in order to develop an interpretive explanation.[4]

Another variant is the "quality circle". This convenes a small group of healthcare providers and patients who meet at regular times for a determined period to formulate hypotheses or action points to improve quality in health care.[5]

Observation based methods

The systematic observation of organisational settings, team behaviour, and interactions is especially useful in studying quality issues as it allows researchers to uncover everyday behaviour rather than relying only on interview accounts. These methods are increasingly used in the study of organisation and delivery of care[6] and can be especially useful in uncovering what really happens in particular healthcare settings – for example, in the study of everyday work in labour wards[7] – and for formative evaluation of new services.

Narrative based medicine

Narrative based medicine is one of several patient centred approaches that can give the physician access to the lived experience of their patients. This is the context in which the physician interprets symptoms and signs and in which personal healthcare decisions are made. It can therefore be an approach to understanding how healthcare decisions are made.

Sampling

Qualitative methods are designed to yield detailed and holistic views of the phenomena under study. The aim of qualitative research is not therefore to identify a statistically representative set of respondents or to produce numerical predictions. Qualitative research questions tend to be exploratory and not tied to formal hypothesis testing, so the sampling strategies used in qualitative research are purposive or theoretical rather than representative or probability based.[8] This means that respondents are sampled based on specific predetermined criteria in order to cover a range of constituencies – for example, different age, social class, and cultural backgrounds (see Box 4.1).[9] To locate hard to reach individuals or groups, researchers can use "convenience" venues, informants, or social networks.

Box 4.1 Focus group study to obtain information directly from adolescent young women on their knowledge and expectations concerning contraceptive use and their attitude to healthcare[9]

To obtain a range of views, a purposive direct sampling strategy was followed to organise the focus groups. Four secondary schools with different educational levels were selected because of the correlation with sexual behaviour of adolescents. In each school all 17 year old young women of one small class were asked to participate. Each group comprised six or seven participants, with a total of 26. Differences in sexual experiences and social classes fostered lively interaction within the groups. The discussions were tape recorded, transcribed, and analysed by content analysis. Knowledge of the daily use and side effects of contraceptives was insufficient. The general practitioner was the most frequently consulted healthcare provider for the first pill prescription, but for a gynaecological examination they thought they had to visit a gynaecologist. Mothers and the peer group were important in teenagers' decision making and should be considered when communicating with adolescent young women.

The sample sizes for interview studies tend to be much smaller than those used in survey or more quantitative research; they may include 30–50 respondents, although this can vary with the research question asked. Similarly, observational studies may be based on a single case study, perhaps focusing on one organisational setting such as a clinic or ward.

Analysis

Qualitative analyses attempt to preserve the textual form of the data gathered and to generate analytical categories and explanations. This may be done inductively – that is, obtained gradually from the data – or deductively – that is, with a theoretical framework as background (Box 4.2),[10] either at the beginning or part way through the analysis as a way of approaching the data.

There are various software packages designed to assist with the organisation and retrieval of qualitative data. Among those most commonly used are QSR NUD*IST[11] and Atlas Ti.[12]

Box 4.2 Investigation of barriers to implementing guidelines for the management of depression in general practice[10]

Information about how general practitioners (34 in the intervention group) managed patients with depression were obtained from review of records and assessment of outcome with a standard patient completed questionnaire. The guidelines were issued to the general practitioners and they were then interviewed individually to identify their personal barriers to acting on the recommendations. The interviews were semi-structured and were recorded and transcribed. Psychological theories of behaviour change were used as the framework for analysing the interviews. The transcripts were repeatedly studied independently by several researchers. An example of the barriers identified through use of a theoretical framework relates to the theory of self-efficacy. Some general practitioners did not feel able to ask about suicide risk because they lacked confidence in their ability to use an appropriate form of words. After the general practitioners had been given suggestions for phrases to use, the proportion of patients whose suicide risk had been assessed increased.

Some of these packages enable sophisticated analysis, allowing the researcher to make theoretical links within the data set; others identify co-occurring codes and provide opportunities to annotate codes or portions of text. All of these processes are integral to qualitative data analysis, but whether software is used or not, the key point about the analysis is that it relies on systematic and rigorous searching of text for categories and themes. These categories and themes are collected together, compared, and re-analysed to develop hypotheses or theoretical explanations. When conducting this coding analysis the researcher gives consideration to the actual words used, the context, the internal consistency, the specificity of responses that is based on the experiences of respondents, and the big ideas beneath all detailed information.[13] It is important in this process not to lose sight of the narrative and textual structure of qualitative data, and to pay attention to the context of items of data (Box 4.3). While software packages can assist with this labour intensive process and offer great potential for managing large data sets, they are not a substitute for thorough knowledge or "immersion" in the data which enables the researcher to identify connections and

Box 4.3 The coding process

(1) As the researcher comes across an idea or phenomenon, a label is attached. A fragment from adolescent girls' focus groups[9]: "*I always talk to my mother because I can tell her everything. You can always get reliable information from your mother.*" Considering the actual words used, possible labels for this fragment are "communication", "mother", "reliable", "information".
(2) When the idea or phenomenon reappears in the text, the label is once again attached. "*If it is really necessary, I will talk to my mother. But I don't like that, but...*"
(3) After reading again all codes and fragments, a better formulation of the code can be found; for this fragment, the label "information sources/mother" can be used.
(4) Specificity: responses based on specific experiences are more important. "*I always talk to my mother. . .*" is more specific than "*Girls of my class are used to talking to their mothers.*"
(5) Codebooks consist of a set of codes that capture the key analytical constructs. Step by step you progress in the level of analysis: raw data → description → interpretation → recommendation.

patterns, to make systematic comparisons, and to develop interpretations.

Reliability and validity

When it comes to judging the quality of qualitative research, qualitative methods are often seen as scoring highly in terms of internal validity. By documenting how people really behave in "natural" everyday situations and examining in detail what people mean when they describe their experiences, feelings, attitudes, and behaviour, these methods are seen as providing an accurate representation of the phenomena studied. Reliability, which is a particular strength of quantitative research, cannot always be judged so easily within a qualitative study. The settings and groups studied within qualitative research may be unique to the particular context or time period, and it is unlikely that a study can be replicated in the way that a controlled experiment can. Sometimes it is possible to involve other researchers in the analytical process to code the data independently or to discuss emerging themes and categories to try to reach consensus about the interpretation of the data. It is important that a clear account of the data collection and analysis is provided to allow readers to judge the evidence and interpretations presented. This clear exposition is also essential for judging the transferability of findings to other settings or groups.

Some examples of qualitative research about the quality of health care

Qualitative research has been used in a number of ways to look at the quality of health care. To illustrate how these methods can inform quality improvement, we focus on three areas where qualitative methods have made a contribution: (1) in identifying salient features of care to inform service delivery and organisation; (2) in exploring organisational and other obstacles to change, notably within the context of healthcare evaluation; and (3) by complementing other research approaches either in the preliminary development of measures or in explaining or implementing findings.

Identifying what really matters to patients and care providers

Interviews or focus group methods are especially helpful in assessing user views of services and healthcare provision and in revealing why some care is perceived as poor quality. One interview study looked at patients' perceptions of the reassurance provided by rheumatologists and found that the typical methods of imparting reassurance, often by minimising or downplaying the seriousness of the arthritic condition, were frequently misinterpreted by patients. This study showed that clinicians needed to be more aware of patients' own views and experience of health problems and to adapt their explanations and information giving to increase its salience for this group of patients.[14] Similarly, an Australian study[15] found that the quality of information and reassurance given to women receiving abnormal cervical smear test results was poor and recommended different ways of organising the service to meet women's information needs and to improve the quality of care.

Qualitative work can be helpful in identifying cultural and social factors that hinder or encourage service use. This information can be directly fed back to healthcare providers to help them improve service delivery (Box 4.1).[9] In the UK, focus groups with women from ethnic minorities[16] identified administrative and language barriers which prevented these women from using cervical screening services.

Identifying obstacles to change

By establishing the reasons behind certain behaviours, qualitative research can help to identify barriers to practice change. Success will be more likely if the methods used to implement change are chosen to address the prevailing barriers.[17] Interview studies have been used to identify modifiable factors associated with prescribing by general practitioners[18] and to distinguish doctor and patient related factors that explain a high level of prescribing of antibiotics.[19] Sometimes qualitative research is helpful in understanding how organisations and teams within them work on a day to day basis. Observational research by Hughes and Griffiths[20] on rationing in cardiac care conferences and neurorehabilitation meetings showed how decisions differed between these two types of service. Making these decision rules explicit makes it possible to see how this process might be improved or adapted. Elsewhere, interviews with general practitioners were used in a randomised trial of the implementation of guidelines for the management of depression in general practice to tailor intervention strategies to the needs of practitioners.[10] The identified barriers to change included doctors' perceived ability to assess suicide risk and inform patients about taking their medication (Box 4.2). Further research is needed to elucidate the most efficient methods for identifying barriers to change and to investigate theoretical frameworks that can be used to understand barriers.

The complex structures and behaviours of healthcare organisations are increasingly recognised as critical factors in determining the quality of care.[21] Qualitative methods offer a potential approach to assisting leaders of organisations to appreciate some of the local issues to be considered when introducing new ideas or transforming systems of care. However, more research is needed to investigate which qualitative methods could be most useful, and in what circumstances they should be used.

Another strength of qualitative research lies in its role within formative evaluation. Qualitative methods can provide insights to the process of policy implementation, identifying where and why this is successful, uncovering initial "teething problems", and suggesting solutions. Qualitative methods have also been used to guide the design of a new "one stop" clinic for women with menstrual problems and to evaluate the service from the patient's perspective.[22]

Complementing other research

Qualitative methods have long been used to inform more quantitative research approaches, notably assisting with research design and the development of outcome measures. They have been used in preliminary work for surveys to develop and test questionnaires – for example, the development of quantitative measures of patients' views should begin with an exploration of the views of samples of patients using qualitative methods (Box 4.4).[23]

Box 4.4 Development of a measure of patients' views of care across the primary/secondary interface[23]

The aim was to develop a standard quantitative measure of the views of patients referred from primary to secondary care. In order to identify the issues of concern to patients, a purposeful sample of patients who had been referred to secondary care was identified. Six focus group meetings were held and five patients who could not travel to a meeting were interviewed individually. Two researchers independently studied the transcripts and developed coding schemes. Differences were resolved through discussion. Five main themes emerged from the data:

- getting into care;
- fitting in with staff and systems of care;
- knowing what's going on (obtaining information);
- continuity of care;
- limbo (progress through the healthcare system).

Failures in the first four themes led patients to report feeling as though they were not making progress and had been left in a state of limbo.

They can also be used as part of the process of dissemination of research evidence, and may be especially helpful in making findings relevant to patients and care providers. Thus, although it can be difficult to incorporate the views of patients or carers, qualitative methods may sometimes be useful in informing recommendations and guidelines.[24,25] The choice of method will depend on the topic and the evidence base, but patient or carer focus groups or interviews can be appropriate if the guideline is concerned with the interpersonal aspects of care, with very small subgroups of patients or carers, or if the available evidence is limited.

Conclusions

This chapter has introduced some of the methods of qualitative research and outlined some ways in which they can contribute to research into quality improvement and management of change. Quality improvement is a major goal of the healthcare systems of most developed countries yet, despite almost two decades of research, effective approaches remain elusive. In order to understand better the human and organisational factors that influence the quality and safety of care, researchers should remember the potential role of qualitative methods. Qualitative research encompasses a range of methods that have successfully been used to explore issues of healthcare delivery from patient and provider perspectives. They can help both to illuminate different facets of "quality" and to inform quantitative approaches to researching health care.

Key messages

- There are several methods for collecting data in qualitative research, including both interview based methods and observation based methods.
- Sampling methods are theoretical or purposive, and analysis may be inductive or deductive.
- These methods may be used to identify what really matters to patients and carers, and can also be used to explain the obstacles to improvement and why improvement does or does not occur.
- Qualitative methods could make an important contribution to understanding how to improve the quality of health care.

Further reading

Suggested introductory books on qualitative research methods:

Denzin NK, Lincoln YS, eds. *Handbook of qualitative research*. Thousand Oaks: Sage, 1998.

Gantley M, Harding G, Kumar S, Tissier J. *An introduction to qualitative methods for health professionals*. Master Classes in Primary Care Research No 1 (Carter Y, Shaw S, Thomas C, eds). London: Royal College of General Practitioners, 1999.

References

1 Strong P, Robinson J. *The NHS: under new management*. Milton Keynes: Open University Press, 1990:81.
2 Mays N, Pope C. Reaching the parts other methods cannot reach: an introduction to qualitative methods in health and health services research. *BMJ* 1995;**311**:42–5.
3 Malterud K. Qualitative research: standards, challenges, and guidelines. *Lancet* 2001;**358**:483–8.
4 Wijnen G, Schillemans L, Hermann I. Introduction of the WVVH prevention card in general practice (in Dutch). *Huisarts Nu* 1993;**22**:17–21.
5 Schillemans L, De Grande L, Remmen R. Using quality circles to evaluate the efficacy of primary health care. In: Conner RF, Hendricks M, eds. *International innovations in evaluation methodology*. New directions in program evaluation 42. San Francisco: Jossey-Bass, 1989:19–27.
6 Murphy E. Micro-level qualitative research. In: Fulop N, Allen P, Clarke A, *et al*, eds. *Studying the organisation and delivery of health services research methods*. London: Routledge, 2001:40–55.
7 Hunt S, Symonds A. *The social meaning of midwifery*. Basingstoke: Macmillan, 1995.
8 Patton M. *Qualitative evaluation and research methods*. Newbury Park, CA: Sage, 1990.
9 Peremans L, Hermann I, Avonts D, *et al*. Contraceptive knowledge and expectations by adolescents: an explanation by focus groups. *Patient Educat Counsel* 2000;**40**:133–41.
10 Baker R, Reddish S, Robertson N, *et al*. Randomised controlled trial of tailored strategies to implement guidelines for the management of patients with depression in general practice. *Br J Gen Pract* 2001;**51**:737–41.
11 Richards T, Richards L. *QSR NUD*IST*. Version 6. London: Sage, 1994.
12 Muhr T. ATLAS/Ti for Windows. Version 4·2. 1996.
13 Krueger RA. *Focus groups. A practical guide for applied research*. London: Sage Publications, 1988.
14 Donovan J, Blake D. Qualitative study of interpretations of reassurance among patients attending rheumatology clinics: "just a touch of arthritis, doctor?" *BMJ* 2000;**320**:541–4.
15 Kavanagh A, Broom D. Women's understanding of abnormal cervical smear test results: a qualitative interview study. *BMJ* 1997;**314**:1388–91.
16 Naish J, Brown J, Denton B. Intercultural consultations: investigation of factors that deter non-English speaking women from attending their general practitioners for cervical screening. *BMJ* 1994;**309**:1126–8.
17 Grol R. Personal paper: beliefs and evidence in changing clinical practice. *BMJ* 1997;**315**:418–21.

18 Carthy P, Harvey I, Brawn R, *et al.* A study of factors associated with cost and variation in prescribing among GPs. *Fam Pract* 2000;**17**:36–41.
19 Coenen S, Van Royen P, Vermeire E, *et al.* Antibiotics for coughing in general practice: a qualitative decision analysis. *Fam Pract* 2000;**17**:380–5.
20 Hughes D, Griffiths L. "Ruling in" and "ruling out": two approaches to the micro rationing of health care. *Soc Sci Med* 1997;**44**:589–99.
21 Plsek P. Redesigning health care with insights from the science of complex adaptive systems. In: Institute of Medicine. *Crossing the quality chasm. A new health system for the 21st century.* Washington DC: National Academy Press, 2001:309–22.
22 Abu J, Baker R, Habiba M, *et al.* Qualitative and quantitative assessment of women's views of a one-stop menstrual clinic compared to traditional gynaecology clinics. *Br J Obstet Gynaecol* 2001;**108**:993–9.
23 Preston C, Cheater F, Baker R, *et al.* Left in limbo: patients' views on care across the primary/secondary interface. *Qual Health Care* 1999;**8**:16–21.
24 Van Wersch A, Eccles M. Involvement of consumers in development of evidence based clinical guidelines: practical experiences from the North of England evidence-based guideline development programme. *Qual Health Care* 2001;**10**:10–16.
25 Katbamna S, Baker R, Ahmad W, *et al.* Development of guidelines to facilitate improved support of South Asian carers by primary health care teams. *Qual Health Care* 2001;**10**:166–72.

5: Research on patients' views in the evaluation and improvement of quality of care

MICHEL WENSING, GLYN ELWYN

The identification of methods for assessing the views of patients on health care has only developed over the last decade or so. The use of patients' views to improve healthcare delivery requires valid and reliable measurement methods. Four approaches are recognised: inclusion of patients' views in the information provided to those seeking health care, identification of patient preferences in episodes of care, patient feedback on delivery of health care, and patients' views in decision making on healthcare systems. Outcome measures for the evaluation of the use of patients' views should reflect the aims in terms of processes or outcomes of care, including possible negative consequences. Rigorous methodologies for the evaluation of methods have yet to be implemented.

Collecting the views of service users has been a key feature of recent developments in society, but it is only over the last decade or so that the healthcare sector has identified methods for assessing the views of patients. A range of methods is available to integrate patients' views on the delivery and improvement of health care, including short questionnaires to assess patients' needs before a consultation with the clinician, focus groups to include patients' views on clinical guidelines, and surveys to provide patient feedback to care providers. If such methods are used for the evaluation and improvement of healthcare systems, they should be studied in terms of effectiveness, efficiency, and maybe even safety.[1] This review shows that this research area has yet to implement rigorous approaches to the collection and synthesis of patients' views.

Table 5.1 Classification of measures of patients' views

	Reports	Ratings
Health status	Functional status measures, measures for disability and handicap; measures of beliefs related to health status (e.g. health locus of control)	Quality of life measures, measures for coping with health problems
Health care	Reports on the use of health care, health care received, and treatment adherence; measures of beliefs related to health care (e.g. efficacy of care providers)	Expectations, needs, preferences, priorities, attitudes, evaluations, complaints, and satisfaction related to health care

Some of the key issues related to the measurement of patients' views and their use in healthcare improvement are considered, together with ways in which the methods themselves may be evaluated.

Measures

Patients' views have different dimensions (Table 5.1). This chapter focuses on patients' views of health care – specifically on their preferences, evaluations, and reports.

Preferences

Preferences are ideas about what should occur in healthcare systems.[2] Related concepts are expectations, perceived needs, desires, wants, requests, and priorities. Expectations have two distinct meanings: beliefs about what should occur or what people want of care ("normative expectations"), and beliefs about what will actually happen, irrespective of whether this is wanted ("predicted expectations").[2] The term "preferences", which has its origins in cognitive psychology and economics, is most often used to refer to individual patients' views about their clinical treatment. The term "priorities" is more often used to describe preferences for healthcare services in a population of patients or citizens.[3] Qualitative as well as quantitative methods can be used to study preferences.

Qualitative research methods such as individual interviews and focus groups can be used to elicit preferences. These methods often use open ended approaches such as topic lists rather than structured questionnaires. It is often difficult for patients to decide what is important in general terms, given the limited experience of any one individual. Focus groups generate interaction among participants which may lead to shared views that transcend individual experiences. It may be helpful to present realistic but hypothetical situations as a trigger for discussions. Facilitation skills may be needed to test whether the group views are well considered and stable.

Quantitative methods for eliciting preferences include surveys and consensus methods such as the Delphi and nominal group techniques. Different types of data can be collected including scale responses that range from "not important" to "extremely important"; rankings – for example, preferences expressed in paired comparisons of alternatives; choice of alternatives – for example, a vote for the most desirable alternatives. Individuals can be asked to rate, rank, or vote for different care providers (GP or hospital) or attributes of care providers – for example, short waiting list, adequate information delivery. In a study of patient priorities in different countries high correlations were found between different methods of rating, ranking of, and voting for aspects of general practice care.[4] A study of different methods for eliciting treatment preferences, however, found significant differences.[5] A range of methods has been developed to collect preference data such as the expectancy value model, multi-attribute utility models, and conjoint analysis models (discrete choice experiments).[6]

A number of methodological issues related to the use of methods for priority setting in health care have been described.[3] A first problem is how "options" are generated: limiting the choices will limit the preference frame. Patients should contribute to the development of a preference framework but they usually lack the expertise to generate a model completely on their own. Decisions in prioritisation issues in healthcare systems inevitably involve a wide array of factors, so methods have to be able to incorporate multidimensional influences. The most realistic methods involve presenting constrained choices where trade-offs have

Box 5.1 Patient preferences for in vitro fertilisation[7]

A conjoint analysis model was developed to predict individuals' preference for receiving different components of an in vitro fertilisation service. Six relevant attributes were identified: chance of taking home a baby, follow up support, time on the waiting list, continuity of staff, cost, and attitudes of staff. Note that these attributes include health outcomes, non-health outcomes, and process attributes. Realistic levels for these attributes were chosen; for instance, "chance of taking home a baby" had the levels 5%, 10%, 15%, 25%, and 35%. A selection of 26 scenarios was chosen (from a possible list of 1000) to achieve a "manageable" option listing for respondents. The 26 scenarios were randomly split into two equal groups and within each group 12 pairwise comparisons were formulated for assessment by randomly selected patients. Regression analysis techniques produced a predictive model of patient preferences for an in vitro fertilisation service. The preferred attributes in this model were staff attitudes, continuity of care, follow up, and chance of taking a baby home.

to be made between different attributes or alternatives. It is important to be explicit about the methods used for the aggregation of individual preferences because different procedures will lead to different results. Researchers should understand that the choice of methods will influence results and should ensure that the assessment processes are at least transparent if methods have the potential to over-represent the views of some population sectors over others. An example of the use of patient preferences is given in Box 5.1.

Evaluations

Patient evaluations are "health care recipients' reactions to salient aspects of the context, process, and result of their service experience".[8] Related concepts are "satisfaction", "unmet needs", "judgements", "complaints", and "comments". The term "evaluation" suggests a cognitive process in which specific aspects of care are assessed, while "satisfaction" refers to an emotional response to the whole experience in health care. The term "patient satisfaction" is probably most often used in the literature.

Many studies have used written questionnaires that comprise structured questions with some sort of rating scale.

The overall satisfaction with the healthcare experience is usually very high and this often masks less positive evaluations when aspects that are more specific are explored. A literature review showed that questionnaires that asked for evaluations in terms of "satisfaction/dissatisfaction" showed less discrimination than questionnaires that used terms such as "good/bad" or "agree/disagree" with very concrete aspects of care.[9] Some questionnaires measure both preferences and experiences and derive evaluations from these two factors by calculating difference or ratio scores.[10] There is some evidence that patients distinguish between the two concepts,[11] but there is no validated framework for deriving evaluations from preferences and experiences.[12]

Patients have evaluative responses to experiences in health care which are not necessarily translated into satisfaction,[13] and qualitative methods can be used to examine these in more depth. An example is shown in Box 5.2. Qualitative approaches are particularly useful for exploring patients' views in areas that have not been fully elaborated. Thorough data analysis of qualitative material is time consuming. Pragmatic approaches such as logging key themes without undertaking full transcription analyses may be used but, as far as we are aware, the reliability and validity of such approaches have not been assessed.

Box 5.2 Patient evaluations of low back pain management[14]

Twenty patients who consulted the general practitioner for low back pain were interviewed shortly after their visit. The general practitioners were also interviewed. A topic list of the key components of a low back pain clinical guideline was used. The data were transcribed and analysed qualitatively. The results revealed that patients often had limited expectations of the consultation. They wanted to hear a diagnosis and expected to receive simple advice. All patients said they complied with the most important advice, which is to stay active, although a few had ideas about possible damage to their back after physical exercise. Patients said they would only take medication if it was strictly necessary, although the guideline recommended analgesics at regular intervals independent of pain. Only one patient demanded physical therapy, although many general practitioners perceived that patients wanted this. Although patients and their general practitioners were satisfied with the chosen management, this study provided deeper understanding of the gap between professional advice and patient motivation to change or act on advice.

Reports

Patient reports represent objective observations of organisation or process of care by patients, regardless of their preferences or evaluations.[15] Patients' experiences and their perceptions of professional performance are similar concepts. Patients can, for instance, register how long they had to wait in the waiting room, irrespective of whether this was too long or not. Although reports reflect patients' observations, they do not necessarily imply a patient's perspective on the quality of care. Nevertheless, patient reports can be used for quality improvement. In some situations patients' reports are the most accurate observation method if, for instance, the data are required about a patient's pathway through different healthcare institutions.

Validity of instruments

Instruments for assessment of patient views of health care should be validated to ensure that the tools measure what they are supposed to measure. A review of 195 studies of patient satisfaction published in 1994 showed that only 89 (46%) reported some validity or reliability data and only 11 (6% of 181 quantitative studies) reported content validity and criterion validity or construct validity and reliability.[16]

Ideally, the instrument should be compared with a gold standard or a criterion measure (an instrument with established validity). For instance, patient reports on the care received can be compared with the medical records or clinicians' reports on the care delivered (Box 5.3). This approach is comparable with the validation of a diagnostic test. A criterion measure for preferences or evaluations is not often available, however, so other approaches are needed.

The validity of most instruments for patients' views should be based on conceptual frameworks that describe a specific domain (the relevant aspects of health care) and it is preferable if patients have been consulted regarding the selection and description of the relevant aspects. Qualitative studies are particularly suitable for that purpose. For instance, the Europep instrument for patients' evaluations of general practice care covers medical care, interpersonal relationships, information and support, and organisation of care. The

Box 5.3 Accuracy of patient reports[15]

Reports of 380 patients obtained through telephone surveys were compared with medical records which were considered to be a gold standard (a disputable perspective as omissions and document loss confound the measures). For chest radiography, mammography, and electrocardiography, patient reports showed high sensitivity and specificity. For serum cholesterol tests, patients proved to be sensitive but not specific reporters. For blood pressure measurements, faecal tests, and rectal examination, false negative rates were below 0·10. They were somewhat higher for breast self-examination instruction and pelvic examination (0·21–0·22). For testicular self-examination instruction patient reports failed to confirm medical record documentation (false negative rate = 0·53).

Box 5.4 Europep instrument[17]

The Europep questionnaire elicits patients' evaluations of general practice care and provides feedback to general practitioners. The originators aimed to develop an instrument that reflected patients' priorities regarding the main areas of general practice care. Validation studies focused on an adequate selection of aspects of care and phrasing of items using a series of systematic evaluations. Literature studies and patient surveys in eight countries were performed to determine these priorities. Preliminary questionnaires were tested in qualitative and quantitative pilot studies. The pre-final 44 item version was formally prepared for international use using forward and backward questionnaire translations. Selection of the final 23 item version was based on the following criteria:

- The questionnaire should cover five main dimensions: interpersonal relationship; medical care; information and support; continuity and cooperation; facilities, availability and accessibility.
- Specific items were included if these referred to aspects of care which were prioritised by patients, showing high item response and reasonable discrimination across patients in most countries. Quantitative cut-off points were defined for these criteria.
- Items were excluded if a serious ambiguity or translation problem was found.

aspects were selected on the basis of literature studies and qualitative and quantitative studies (Box 5.4).

Sometimes it is possible to verify whether patients' views are associated with other factors or whether the measure meets criteria set by the theory from which the measure has been derived (construct validity). For instance, most patient satisfaction studies have shown that older patients have more positive evaluations of health care than younger patients. It can therefore be predicted that a new measure for patient satisfaction will show similar associations.

Psychometrics

Quantitative instruments should have adequate psychometric features.[18] High item response rates will indicate the presence of questions that are more likely to be relevant and understandable. Some instruments, however, are intended to identify rare events such as medical errors (complaint procedures) or side effects of medications (surveys among drug users). High item response rates are not relevant in such cases. Instruments designed to measure aspects of quality should also show good variation across patients (discrimination) and variation between measurements at different points in time (responsiveness). If indicators are supposed to be clustered within dimensions, validity is supported by proven unidimensionality and high internal consistency. However, not all instruments assume clustering between indicators because indicators may not be seen as repeated measurements. This will be the case for many instruments that measure reports of concrete aspects of care. Ideally, instruments will also show good test–retest reliability.

The most often used reliability coefficients refer to the internal consistency of items within a dimension per patient – for example, Cronbach's alpha. In the context of quality improvement, however, aggregated scores per care provider are often needed – that is, aggregation over many individuals. These figures are based on a number of indicators and a number of patients or events. An example is the percentage of patients with positive evaluations of the accessibility of care in a specific hospital based on a survey of 100 patients who answered 10 different questions on accessibility. Generalisability analyses can be used to calculate reliability coefficients for the aggregated scores.[19] It appears that an increase in the number of patients often has more influence on the reliability of the aggregated scores than an increase in the number of indicators.

Sampling

The inclusion criteria for the study population determine the generalisability or external validity of a study or audit. For instance, measurements among patients who attend a clinician are not generalisable to the general patient population registered at a practice or a population of Internet users who visit a site on a health problem. Qualitative studies use theoretical sampling to achieve a specific sample which may be heterogeneous or homogeneous, depending on the overall purpose of the work. Quantitative studies use many different forms of sampling methods to achieve a representative sample (random, stratified, etc). It is important to achieve high response rates and low dropouts in order to avoid selection bias (except if this was sought). Non-responders are more likely to be represented by those who are ill, less satisfied with care provided, and less frequent users of health care than responders.[20,21] Surveys of interview methods need to consider the impact in case these groups are excluded or drop out.

Response rates in surveys among patients vary considerably. A literature review reported a mean of 60% in response rates and a standard deviation of 21%.[22] Many factors may influence the response rate of a survey, such as the motivation of the clinician to recruit patients, the attractiveness of the layout of a questionnaire, the method of administering the questionnaire to patients, the use of monetary incentives, and possibly the use of information technology for administering questionnaires. Insight into which factors are most relevant is limited. A comparison of handing out questionnaires to visitors to the general practice and mailing questionnaires to patients at home gave response rates of 72% and 63%, respectively; the content of the answers of both sample populations was, however, largely similar.[23] A randomised trial showed that written reminders could improve the response rates unless the rate was already above 80%.[24]

Use of patients' views for quality improvement

Table 5.2 outlines the potential use of patients' views in healthcare delivery and quality improvement.[25] One approach

Table 5.2 Use of patients' views for quality improvement

Provision of data to those who seek health care:
- Health education
- Internet communication
- Public reports

Eliciting patient preferences in episodes of care:
- Needs assessment
- Tailored patient education
- Shared decision making
- Patient-held records

Patients' feedback on medical care:
- Written surveys
- Complaint procedures
- Patient participation groups

Patient involvement in healthcare systems:
- Assessment of priorities
- Involvement in guidelines
- Patient organisations

focuses on those who want to make choices about their utilisation of healthcare services. Health education materials may include information on patients' views based, for instance, on qualitative research of their experiences in health care. Public reports on the performance of different care providers may include information about patients' evaluations of care.[26] A comparison with other care providers requires adequate adjustment for case mix, which is difficult because insight into predictors of patient evaluations of care (and most other indicators) is limited.[26]

Another approach focuses on patients in episodes of care using, for instance, shared decision making strategies or patient-held records. Identification of patient preferences is part of most of these approaches. For instance, shared decision making implies that the care provider gives information on relevant options, assesses patient preferences regarding these options, and takes a decision with or checks approval of the patient.[27] A third approach provides different types of patient feedback on health care received derived from surveys, patient groups, or complaint procedures. These views can be used for continuing education and service improvements. Patient views can be compared with ethical or clinical guidelines for

Table 5.3 Objectives of patient involvement and relevant measures

Objectives	Relevant measures
Adhere to ethical principles	Assess the impact of the processes of involvement at different levels (service design, clinical interactions, feedback systems) with criteria derived from ethical principles
Meet patients' preferences	Same as above, but with patient-based criteria
Provide improved care process	Assess doctor–patient communication, medical care, organisation of care, etc.
Provide improved patient outcomes	Assess patient compliance, health status, anxiety, coping, satisfaction with care, etc.
Achieve political or strategic aims	Assess the position on healthcare market, democratic organisation, etc.

good practice but, in many cases, such standards are difficult to define. An exception is a lawsuit where an ethical or legal assessment is explicitly sought. Comparison with other care providers can help to prioritise issues that need attention.

A fourth approach focuses on the involvement of patients and the public in the design and planning of healthcare systems. This requires information on patients' views such as studies of patient priorities or the assessment of local needs for health care. Patient organisations express the views of patients who coalesce around issues or conditions and these may differ from the aggregated views of individuals in wider populations. In these situations, patients' views are only one of a number of inputs into a wider policy making process.

Relevant outcomes

Methods to identify and use patients' views for the improvement of health care can be seen as a technology which should be evaluated in terms of effectiveness and efficiency. The choice of relevant outcomes for the use of patients' views for quality improvement requires further attention. It appears logical to derive outcome measures for the evaluation from the underlying objectives of this effort (Table 5.3).

It is an ethical and legal rule that patients should be informed and involved in their health care, at least to minimal standards. Many patients wish to be involved in the decision processes, at least to some extent.[28] In line with this aim, the process of involvement rather than its outcome is crucial and so it is the ethical principles and patient preferences that define the criteria for effectiveness. For instance, shared decision making can be evaluated in terms of information delivered on treatment options, checking of understanding and preferences, and making a shared decision.[29]

Patient involvement may also result in better processes and outcomes of care. It could, for instance, make clinicians more responsive to patient preferences, contribute to a better implementation of clinical guidelines, and result in better adherence to treatment, health status, and satisfaction with care. Patients can be seen as co-producers of health care because their decisions and behaviour influence healthcare provision and its outcomes. Outcome measures should reflect the effects on process or outcomes of care that are expected.

Integration of patients' views may be driven by political and strategic motivations such as protection of a position in a competitive healthcare market, the wish to have democratic control in the healthcare organisation, or the need to do something for underserved populations. Such aims may be difficult to assess, but measurable outcome measures can be found in some cases – for instance, position on the healthcare market can be evaluated in terms of attendance rates and turnover of patients.

Finally, evaluations should consider possible negative consequences such as unrealistic patient expectations of what health care can deliver; defensive behaviour of care providers, resulting in higher numbers of unnecessary clinical procedures; undermining of professional morale; and increased costs. Such consequences are not imaginary. A randomised trial on low back pain showed that 80% would have chosen radiography if available, but that patients who received radiography often had more pain at three months than the control group and were nevertheless more satisfied with the care provided.[30]

Not only should the effects of specific methods be studied, but also their actual uptake in health care. Clinicians and patients may lack competence or skills to use specific instruments or have negative attitudes regarding specific approaches. Organisational structures may limit the application of specific methods. Such barriers need to be identified and addressed by means of targeted strategies which should be evaluated in terms of success of uptake of the methods.

Conclusions

A range of approaches is available to integrate patients' views into healthcare delivery systems and their improvement. The methods to measure and use patients' views should be studied in the context of their intended application. Quantitative as well as qualitative approaches can be used to measure patients' views, and the validity and reliability of the methods should be examined. The effectiveness and efficiency of the methods should be studied in terms of their consequences for process and outcomes of health care. Increased patient participation in health care can be seen as desirable in itself, but this should not inhibit evaluation of the methods used to achieve this aim.

Key messages

- Patients' views include preferences (ideas about what should occur), evaluations (judgements of aspects of care), and reports (observations of organisation or process of care).
- The validity of measures of patients' views should be based on conceptual frameworks, preferably derived from rigorous qualitative studies.
- Effective methods for reporting information on patients' views are needed to influence and improve process and outcomes within healthcare systems.

References

1 Wensing M. Evidence-based patient empowerment (editorial). *Qual Health Care* 2000;**9**:200–1.
2 Uhlmann RF, Inui TS, Carter WB. Patient requests and expectations. Definitions and clinical applications. *Med Care* 1984;**22**:681–5.
3 Mullen PM. Public involvement in health care priority setting: an overview of methods for eliciting values. *Health Expect* 1999;**2**:222–34.

4 Grol R, Wensing M, Mainz J, *et al*. Patients' priorities with respect to general practice care: an international comparison. *Fam Pract* 1999;**16**:4–11.
5 Souchek J, Stacks JR, Brody B, *et al*. A trial for comparing methods for eliciting treatment preferences from men with advanced prostate cancer. Results from the initial visit. *Med Care* 2000;**38**:1040–50.
6 Froberg DG, Kane RL. Methodology for measuring health-state preferences – 1: Measurement strategies. *J Clin Epidemiol* 1989;**42**:345–54.
7 Ryan M. Using conjoint analysis to take account of patient preferences and go beyond health outcomes: an application to in vitro fertilisation. *Soc Sci Med* 1999;**48**:535–46.
8 Pascoe GC. Patient satisfaction in primary health care: a literature review and analysis. *Eval Program Planning* 1983;**6**:185–210.
9 Wensing M, Grol R, Smits A. Quality judgements by patients on general practice care: a literature analysis. *Soc Sci Med* 1994;**38**:45–53.
10 Sixma HJ, Van Campen C, Kerssens JJ, *et al*. Quality of care from the perspective of elderly people: the QUOTE-Elderly instrument. *Age Ageing* 2000;**29**:173–8.
11 Jung HP, Wensing M, Grol R. Comparison of patients' preferences and evaluations regarding aspects of general practice care. *Fam Pract* 2000;**17**:236–42.
12 Baker R. Pragmatic model of patient satisfaction in general practice: progress towards a theory. *Qual Health Care* 1997;**6**:201–4.
13 Williams B. Patient satisfaction: a valid concept? *Soc Sci Med* 1994;**38**:509–16.
14 Schers H, Wensing M, Huijsmans S, *et al*. Low back pain management in primary care. *Spine* 2001;**26**:E348–53.
15 Brown JB, Adams ME. Patients as reliable reporters of medical care process. Recall of ambulatory encounter events. *Med Care* 1992;**30**: 400–11.
16 Sitzia J. How valid and reliable are patient satisfaction data? An analysis of 195 studies. *Int J Qual Health Care* 1999;**11**:319–28.
17 Grol R, Wensing M, for the Europep Group. *Patients evaluate general/family practice: the Europep instrument*. Nijmegen: Wonca/EQuiP, 2000.
18 Streiner DL, Norman GR. *Health measurement scales. A practical guide to their development and use*. Oxford: Oxford University Press, 1989.
19 O'Brien RM. Generalizability coefficients are reliability coefficients. *Qual Quant* 1995;**29**:421–8.
20 Rubin HR. Can patients evaluate the quality of hospital care? *Med Care Rev* 1990;**47**:267–325.
21 Etter JF, Perneger TV. Analysis of non-response bias in a mailed health survey. *J Clin Epidemiol* 1997;**50**:1123–8.
22 Asch DA, Jedrziewski MK, Christakis NA. Response rates to mail surveys published in medical journals. *J Clin Epidemiol* 1997;**50**:1129–36.
23 Wensing M, Grol R, Smits A, *et al*. Evaluation of general practice care by chronically ill patients: effect of the method of administration. *Fam Pract* 1996;**13**:386–90.
24 Wensing M, Mainz J, Kvamme O, *et al*. Effect of mailed reminders on the response rate in surveys among patients in general practice. *J Clin Epidemiol* 1999;**52**:585–7.
25 Wensing M, Grol R. What can patients do to improve health care? *Health Expect* 1998;**1**:37–49.
26 Marshall MN, Shekelle PG, Leatherman S, *et al*. Public disclosure of performance data: learning from the US experience. *Qual Health Care* 2000;**9**:53–7.

27 Elwyn G, Edwards A, Kinnersley P, *et al.* Shared decision-making and the concept of equipoise: defining the competences of involving patients in healthcare choices. *Br J Gen Pract* 2000;**50**:892–9.
28 Guadagnoli E, Ward P. Patient participation in decision-making. *Soc Sci Med* 1998;**47**:329–39.
29 Edwards A, Elwyn G. How should effectiveness of risk communication to aid patients' decisions to be judged? A review of the literature. *Med Decision Making* 1999;**19**:428–34.
30 Kendrick D, Fielding K, Bentley E, *et al.* Radiography of the lumbar spine in primary care patients with low back pain: randomised trial. *BMJ* 2001;**322**:400–5.

6: Systematic reviews of the effectiveness of quality improvement strategies and programmes

JEREMY GRIMSHAW, LAURA M MCAULEY,
LISA A BERO, ROBERTO GRILLI,
ANDREW D OXMAN, CRAIG RAMSAY,
LUKE VALE, MERRICK ZWARENSTEIN

Systematic reviews provide the best evidence on the effectiveness of healthcare interventions including quality improvement strategies. The methods of systematic review of individual patient randomised trials of healthcare interventions are well developed. We discuss methodological and practice issues that need to be considered when undertaking systematic reviews of quality improvement strategies including developing a review protocol, identifying and screening evidence sources, quality assessment and data abstraction, analytical methods, reporting systematic reviews, and appraising systematic reviews. This chapter builds on our experiences within the Cochrane Effective Practice and Organisation of Care (EPOC) review group.

Systematic reviews are "reviews of a clearly formulated question that use explicit methods to identify, select, and critically appraise relevant research and to collect and analyse data from the studies that are included in the review".[1] Well conducted systematic reviews are increasingly seen as providing the best evidence to guide choice of quality improvement strategies in health care.[2–4] Furthermore, systematic reviews should be an integral part of the planning of future quality improvement research to ensure that the proposed research is informed by all relevant current research and that the research questions have not already been answered.

Systematic reviews are a generic methodology that can be used to synthesise evidence from a broad range of methods addressing different types of questions (Box 6.1). Mulrow[6] suggested that, in comparison with traditional narrative reviews, systematic reviews are an efficient scientific approach to identify and summarise evidence on the effectiveness of interventions that allow the generalisability and consistency of research findings to be assessed and data inconsistencies to be explored. Furthermore, the explicit methods used in systematic reviews should limit bias and improve the reliability and accuracy of conclusions. In this chapter we focus on the methods of systematic reviews of the effectiveness of quality improvement strategies and programmes, building on our experiences within the Cochrane Effective Practice and Organisation of Care (EPOC) review group (Box 6.2).[7–9] (For a more general discussion about the conduct of systematic reviews see the Cochrane Handbook,[10] Egger and colleagues,[11] and Cooper and Hedges.[12])

Forming a review team

When preparing to undertake a systematic review of a quality improvement strategy it is important to assemble a review team with the necessary combination of content and technical expertise. Content expertise may come from consumers, healthcare professionals, and policy makers. Content expertise is necessary to ensure that the review question is sensible and addresses the concerns of key stakeholders, and to aid interpretation of the review. Frequently, content experts may not have adequate technical expertise and require additional support during the conduct of reviews. Technical expertise is required to develop search strategies for major databases, hand search key journals (when appropriate), screen search results, develop data abstraction forms, appraise quality of primary studies, and statistically pool data (when appropriate).

Box 6.1 Steps involved in undertaking a systematic review

- Stating the objectives of the research
- Defining eligibility criteria for studies to be included
- Identifying (all) potentially eligible studies
- Applying eligibility criteria
- Assembling the most complete data set feasible
- Analysing this data set, using statistical synthesis and sensitivity analyses, if appropriate and possible
- Preparing a structured report of the research

From Chalmers[5]

Box 6.2 The Cochrane Effective Practice and Organisation of Care (EPOC) Group

The Cochrane Effective Practice and Organisation of Care (EPOC) group undertakes systematic reviews of the effectiveness of professional, organisational, financial, and regulatory interventions to improve professional practice and the delivery of effective health services.[6–8] It was established in 1994 and since then has worked with over 180 reviewers worldwide to produce 29 reviews and 22 protocols covering a diverse range of topics including the effectiveness of different continuing medical education strategies, changes in the setting of care and different remuneration systems for primary care physicians.

Developing a protocol for a systematic review

Before undertaking a systematic review it is important to develop a formal protocol detailing the background, objectives, inclusion criteria, search methods, and proposed analytical methods to be used in the review. If reviewers do not develop a protocol a priori, there is a danger that the results of the review may be influenced by the data. For example, reviewers may exclude studies with unexpected or undesirable results.[13] Developing and following a detailed protocol protects against this potential bias. Examples of protocols for reviews of quality improvement strategies are available in The Cochrane Library and from the EPOC website.[8,9]

Inclusion criteria for systematic reviews

Reviewers need to develop the review question based upon consideration of the types of study (for example, randomised controlled trials), interventions (for example, audit and feedback), study populations (for example, physicians), and outcomes (for example, objective measures of provider behaviour) in which they are interested. In general it is better to choose an estimation approach rather than a hypothesis testing approach in systematic reviews of quality improvement strategies as decision makers want to know something about the size of the expected effects (and the uncertainty around those estimates), and not just whether the null hypothesis can be rejected or not. Moreover, focusing on hypothesis testing tends to focus attention on p values rather than effects.

It is often helpful for reviewers to attempt to frame their research question in terms of the effects of quality improvement strategy *x* on end point *y* in study population *z*. In addition, reviewers should attempt to define a priori any subgroup analyses they wish to undertake to explore effect modifiers (for example, characteristics of the intervention) or other sources of heterogeneity (for example, quality of the included studies).

Design considerations

While cluster randomised trials are the most robust design for quality improvement strategies,[13] some strategies may not be amenable to randomisation – for example, mass media campaigns. Under these circumstances, reviewers may choose to include other designs including quasi-experimental designs.[14] If a review includes quasi-experimental studies – for example, interrupted time series designs for evaluating mass media campaigns,[15] the reviewers need to recognise the weaknesses of such designs and be cautious of overinterpreting the results of such studies. Within EPOC, reviewers can include randomised trials, controlled before and after studies, and interrupted time series.[8]

Intervention considerations

Another important issue faced by reviewers is the lack of generally accepted classification of quality improvement strategies; as a result, it is vital that reviewers clearly define the intervention of interest. In our experience it is easier to define interventions based on pragmatic descriptions of the components of an intervention – for example, interactive educational sessions – than theoretical constructs – for example, problem based learning – as the description of interventions in primary studies is commonly poorly reported, especially lacking details of the rationale or theoretical basis for an intervention. Developing the definition of an intervention that can be operationalised within a systematic review frequently requires several iterations, preferably with involvement of content experts outside the review team to ensure that the resulting definitions are likely to be robust and meaningful. EPOC has developed a taxonomy for quality improvement interventions based on such descriptions that may provide a useful starting point for such discussions (see Box 6.3 for examples).

The lumping versus splitting debate

A key issue faced by reviewers of quality improvement strategies is deciding how broad the scope of a review should be; this is commonly know as the "lumping" or "splitting" debate.[17] For example, a review team could choose to undertake a review of quality improvement interventions to improve chronic diseases across all healthcare settings and professionals, or a review of quality improvement interventions to improve chronic diseases within primary care, or a review of quality improvement strategies to improve diabetes care within primary care, or a review of audit and feedback to improve all aspects of care across all healthcare settings. The rationale for taking a broad approach ("lumping") is that, because systematic reviews aim to identify the common generalisable features within similar interventions, minor differences in study characteristics may not be crucially important. The rationale for taking a narrower approach ("splitting") is that it is only appropriate to include studies which are very similar in design, study population, intervention characteristics, and outcome recording.

There are good methodological reasons for taking a broad approach. Broad systematic reviews allow the generalisability and consistency of research findings to be assessed across a wider range of different settings, study populations, and

Box 6.3 Examples from the EPOC taxonomy of professional quality improvement strategies[16]

- Distribution of educational materials: published or printed recommendations for clinical care including clinical practice guidelines, delivered personally or through mass mailings.
- Educational meetings: healthcare providers who have participated in conferences, lectures, workshops, or traineeships.
- Local consensus processes: inclusion of participating providers in discussion to ensure that they agreed that the chosen clinical problem was important and the approach to managing the problem was appropriate.
- Educational outreach visits and academic detailing: use of a trained person who met with providers in their practice settings to give information with the intent of changing the provider's practice. The information given may have included feedback on the performance of the provider(s).
- Local opinion leaders: use of providers nominated by their colleagues as "educationally influential". The investigators must have explicitly stated that their colleagues identified the opinion leaders.
- Patient mediated interventions: new clinical information (not previously available) collected directly from patients and given to the provider – e.g. depression scores from an instrument.
- Audit and feedback: any summary of clinical performance of health care over a specified period of time. The summary may also have included recommendations for clinical action. The information may have been obtained from medical records, computerised databases, or observations from patients.
- Reminders: patient or encounter specific information, provided verbally, on paper, or on a computer screen, which is designed or intended to prompt a health professional to recall information, including computer aided decision support and drug dosage information.
- Marketing: a survey of targeted providers to identify barriers to change and subsequent design of an intervention that addresses identified barriers.

behaviours. This reduces the risk of bias or chance results. For example, Jamtvedt and colleagues undertook a review of audit and feedback to improve all aspects of care across all healthcare settings.[18] They identified 85 studies of which 18 considered the effects of audit and feedback on chronic disease management, 14 considered the effects of audit and feedback on chronic disease management in primary care, and three considered the effects of audit and feedback on diabetes care in primary care settings. By undertaking a broad review they were able to explore whether the effects of audit and feedback were similar across different types of behaviour, different settings, and different types of behaviour within different settings. If they had undertaken a narrow review of audit and feedback on diabetes care in primary care they would have been limited to considering only three studies and may have made erroneous conclusions if these studies suffered from bias or chance results. Very narrowly focused reviews are, in effect, subgroup analyses and suffer all the well recognised potential hazards of such analyses.[19] A more transparent approach is to lump together all similar interventions and then to carry out explicit a priori subgroup analyses.

Identifying and screening evidence sources

Reviewers need to identify what bibliographic databases and other sources the review team will search to identify potentially relevant studies, and the proposed search strategies for the different databases. There is a wide range of bibliographic databases available – for example, Medline, Embase, CINAHL, PsycLIT, ERIC, SIGLE. The review team has to make a judgement about what databases are most relevant to the review question and can be searched within the resources available to them.

The review team has to develop sensitive search strategies for potentially relevant studies. Unfortunately, quality improvement strategies are poorly indexed within bibliographic databases: as a result, broad search strategies using free text and allied MeSH headings often need to be used. Furthermore, while optimal search strategies have been developed for identifying randomised controlled trials,[20] efficient search strategies have not been developed for quasi-experimental designs. Review teams should include or consult with experienced information scientists to provide technical expertise in this area.

EPOC has developed a highly sensitive search strategy (available at http://www.epoc.uottawa.ca/register.htm) for studies within its scope, and has searched Medline, Embase,

CINAHL and SIGLE retrospectively and prospectively.[21] We have screened over 200 000 titles and abstracts retrieved by our searches of these databases to identify potentially relevant studies. These are entered onto a database ("pending") awaiting further assessment of the full text of the paper. Studies which, after this assessment, we believe to be within our scope are then entered onto our database (the "specialised register") with hard copies kept in our editorial base. We currently have approximately 2500 studies in our specialised register (with a further 3000 potentially relevant studies currently being assessed). In future, reviewers may wish to consider the EPOC specialised register as their main bibliographic source for reviews and only undertake additional searches if the scope of their review is not within EPOC's scope (see EPOC website for further information about the register).[9]

Preferably two reviewers should independently screen the results of searches and assess potentially relevant studies against the inclusion criteria in the protocol. The reasons for excluding potentially relevant studies should be noted when the review is reported.

Quality assessment and data abstraction

Studies meeting the inclusion criteria should be assessed against quality criteria. While there is growing empirical evidence about sources of bias in individual patient randomised trials of healthcare interventions,[22] quality criteria for cluster randomised trials and quasi experimental are less developed. EPOC has developed quality appraisal criteria for such studies based upon threats to validity of such studies identified by Cook and Campbell[23] (available from the EPOC website).[9] Reviewers should develop a data abstraction checklist to ensure a common approach is applied across all studies. Box 6.4 provides examples of data abstraction checklist items that reviewers may wish to collect. Data abstraction should preferably be undertaken independently by two reviewers. The review team should identify the methods that will be used to resolve disagreements.

Box 6.4 Examples of data abstraction checklist items

- Inclusion criteria
- Type of targeted behaviour
- Participants
  - Characteristics of participating providers
  - Characteristics of participating patients
- Study setting
  - Location of care
  - Country
- Study methods
  - Unit of allocation/analysis
  - Quality criteria
- Prospective identification by investigators of barriers to change
- Type and characteristics of interventions
  - Nature of desired change
  - Format/sources/recipient/method of delivery/timing
- Type of control intervention (if any)
- Outcomes
  - Description of the main outcome measure(s)
- Results

Derived from EPOC data abstraction checklist[8,16]

Preparing for data analysis

The methodological quality of primary studies of quality improvement strategies is often poor. Reviewers frequently need to make decisions about which outcomes to include within data analyses and may need to undertake re-analysis of some studies. In this section we highlight methods for addressing two common problems encountered in systematic reviews of quality improvement strategies – namely, reporting of multiple end points and handling unit of analysis errors in cluster randomised studies.

Reporting multiple outcomes

Commonly, quality improvement studies report multiple end points – for example, changes in practice for 10 different preventive services or diagnostic tests. While reviewers may choose to report all end points, this is problematic both for the analysis and for readers who may be overwhelmed with data. The review team should decide which end points it will report and include in the analysis. For example, a review team could choose to use the main end points specified by the investigators when this is done, and the median end point when the main end points are not specified.[21]

Handling unit of analysis errors in primary studies

Many cluster randomised trials have potential unit of analysis errors; practitioners or healthcare organisations are randomised but during the statistical analyses the individual patient data are analysed as if there was no clustering within practitioner or healthcare organisation.[14,24] In a recent systematic review of guideline dissemination and implementation strategies over 50% of included cluster randomised trials had such unit of analysis errors.[21] Potential unit of analysis errors result in artificially low p values and overly narrow confidence intervals.[25] It is possible to re-analyse the results of cluster randomised trials if a study reports event rates for each of the clusters in the intervention and control groups using a *t* test, or if a study reports data on the extent of statistical clustering.[25,26] In our experience it is rare for studies with unit of analysis errors to report sufficient data to allow re-analysis. The point estimate is not affected by unit of analysis errors, so it is possible to consider the size of the effects reported in these studies even though the statistical significance of the results cannot be ascertained (see Donner and Klar[27] for further discussion on systematic reviews of clustered data and Grimshaw and colleagues[20] and Ramsay and colleagues[28] for further discussion of other common methodological problems in primary studies of quality improvement strategies).

Methods of analysis/synthesis

Meta-analysis

When undertaking systematic reviews it is often possible to undertake meta-analyses that use "statistical techniques within a systematic review to integrate the results of individual studies".[1] Meta-analyses combine data from multiple studies and summarise all the reviewed evidence by a single statistic, typically a pooled relative risk of an adverse outcome with confidence intervals. Meta-analysis assumes that different studies addressing the same issue will tend to have findings in the same direction.[29] In other words, the *real* effect of an intervention may vary in magnitude but will be in the same direction. Systematic reviews of quality improvement strategies typically include studies that exhibit greater variability or *heterogeneity* of estimates of effectiveness of such interventions due to differences in how interventions were operationalised, targeted behaviours, targeted professionals, and study contexts. As a result, the real effect of an intervention may vary both in magnitude and in direction, depending on the modifying effect of such factors. Under these circumstances, meta-analysis may result in an artificial result which is potentially misleading and of limited value to decision makers. Further reports of primary studies frequently have common methodological problems – for example, unit of analysis errors – or do not report data necessary for meta-analysis. Given these considerations, many existing reviews of quality improvement strategies have used qualitative synthesis methods rather than meta-analysis.

Although deriving an average effect across a heterogeneous group of studies is unlikely to be helpful, quantitative analyses can be useful for describing the range and distribution of effects across studies and to explore probable explanations for the variation that is found. Generally, a combination of quantitative analysis, including visual analyses, and qualitative analysis should be used.

Qualitative synthesis methods

Previous qualitative systematic reviews of quality improvement strategies have largely used vote counting methods that add up the number of positive and negative comparisons and conclude whether the interventions were effective on this basis.[2,30] Vote counting can count either the number of comparisons with a positive direction of effect (irrespective of statistical significance) or the number of comparisons with statistically significant effects. These approaches suffer from a number of weaknesses. Vote counting comparisons with a positive direction fail to provide an estimate of the effect size of an intervention (giving equal weight to comparisons that show a 1% change or a 50% change) and ignore the precision of the estimate from the primary comparisons (giving equal weight to comparisons with 100 or 1000 participants). Vote counting comparisons with statistically significant effects suffer similar problems; in addition, comparisons with potential unit of analysis errors need to be excluded because of the uncertainty about their statistical significance, and underpowered comparisons observing clinically significant but statistically insignificant effects would be counted as "no effect comparisons".

To overcome some of these problems, we have been exploring more explicit analytical approaches, reporting:

- the number of comparisons showing a positive direction of effect
- the median effect size across all comparisons
- the median effect size across comparisons without unit of analysis errors; and
- the number of comparisons showing statistically significant effects.[21]

This allows the reader to assess the likely effect size and consistency of effects across all included studies and whether these effects differ between studies, with and without unit of analysis errors. By using these more explicit methods we are able to include information from all studies, but do not have the same statistical certainty of the effects as we would using a vote counting approach. An example of the impact of this approach is shown in Box 6.5.

Exploring heterogeneity

When faced with heterogeneity in both quantitative and qualitative systematic reviews, it is important to explore the potential causes of this in a narrative and statistical manner (where appropriate).[32] Ideally, the review team should have identified potential effect modifiers a priori within the review protocol. It is possible to explore heterogeneity using tables, bubble plots, and whisker plots (displaying medians, interquartile ranges, and ranges) to compare the size of the observed effects in relationship to each of these modifying variables.[18] Meta-regression is a multivariate statistical

Box 6.5 Impact of using an explicit analytical approach

Freemantle et al[31] used a vote counting approach in a review of the effects of disseminating printed educational materials. None of the studies using appropriate statistical analyses found statistically significant improvements in practice. The authors concluded: "This approach has led researchers and quality improvement professionals to discount printed educational materials as possible interventions to improve care".

In contrast, Grimshaw et al[21] used an explicit analytical approach in a review of the effects of guideline dissemination and implementation strategies. Across four cluster randomised controlled trials they observed a median absolute improvement of +8·1% (range +3·6% to +17%) compliance with guidelines. Two studies had potential unit of analysis errors, the remaining two studies observed no statistically significant effects. They concluded: "These results suggest that educational materials may have a modest effect on guideline implementation ... However the evidence base is sparse and of poor quality". This approach, by capturing more information, led to the recognition that printed educational materials may result in modest but important improvements in care and required further evaluation.

technique that can be used to examine how the observed effect sizes are related to potential explanatory variables. However, the small number of included studies common in systematic review of quality improvement strategies may lead to overfitting and spurious claims of association. Furthermore, it is important to recognise that these associations are observational and may be confounded by other factors.[33] As a result, such analyses should be seen as exploratory. Graphical presentation of such analyses often facilitates understanding as it allows several levels of information to be conveyed concurrently (Figure 6.1).

This bubble plot, from a review on the effects of audit and feedback,[18] shows the relationship between the adjusted risk difference and baseline non-compliance. The adjusted risk difference represents the difference in non-compliance before the intervention from the difference observed after the intervention. Each bubble represents a study, and the size of the bubble reflects the number of healthcare providers in the study. The regression line shows a trend towards increased compliance with audit and feedback with increasing baseline non-compliance.

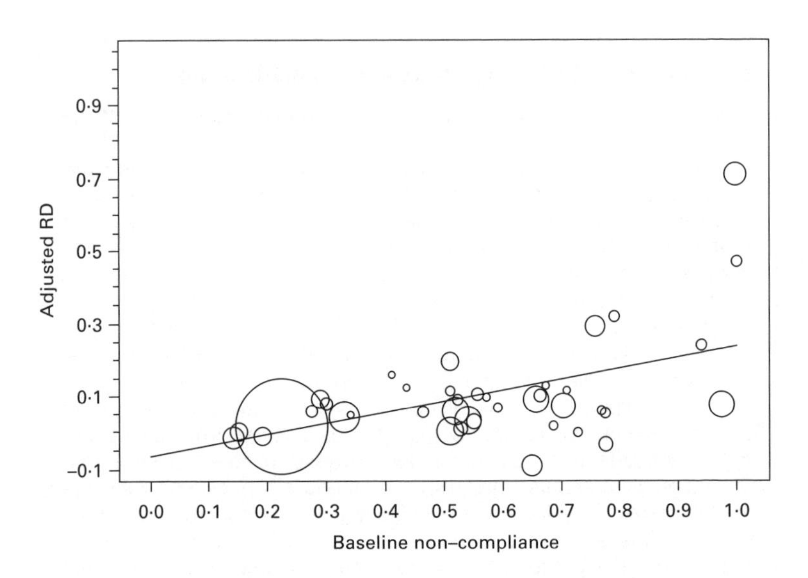

Figure 6.1 Graphical presentation of results using a bubble plot

Appraising systematic reviews of quality improvement strategies

Systematic reviews of quality improvement strategies are of varying quality and potential users of such reviews should appraise their quality carefully. Fortunately, Oxman and colleagues have developed and validated a checklist for appraising systematic reviews including nine criteria scored as "done", "partially done", and "not done", and one summary criterion scored on a 1–7 scale where 1 indicates "major risk of bias" and 7 indicates "minor risk of bias" (Box 6.6).[34,35] Grimshaw and colleagues used this scale to appraise 41 systematic reviews of quality improvement strategies published by 1998; the median summary quality score was 4, indicating that they had some methodological flaws.[3] Common methodological problems within these reviews included failure to adequately report inclusion criteria, to avoid bias in the selection of studies, to report criteria to assess the validity of included studies; and failure to apply criteria to assess the

Box 6.6 Checklist for appraising systematic reviews

(1) Were the search methods used to find evidence (primary studies) on the primary question(s) stated?
(2) Was the search for evidence reasonably comprehensive?
(3) Were the criteria used for deciding which studies to include in the review reported?
(4) Was bias in the selection of articles avoided?
(5) Were the criteria used for assessing the validity of the studies that were reviewed reported?
(6) Was the validity of all the studies referred to in the text assessed using appropriate criteria (either in selecting studies for inclusion or in analysing the studies that are cited)?
(7) Were the methods used to combine the findings of the relevant studies (to reach a conclusion) reported?
(8) Were the findings of the relevant studies combined appropriately relative to the primary question addressed by the review?
(9) Were the conclusions made by the author(s) supported by the data and/or the analysis reported in the review?
(10) Overall, how would you rate the scientific quality of this review?

Items 1–9 scored as done, not clear, not done.
Item 10 scored on a scale of 1 (major risk of bias) to 7 (minimal risk of bias).
Adapted from Oxman[34] and Oxman and Guyatt.[35]

validity of selected studies. Unit of analysis errors were rarely addressed in these reviews.

Conclusion

Systematic reviews are increasingly recognised as the best evidence source on the effectiveness of different quality improvement strategies. In this paper we have discussed issues that reviewers face when conducting reviews of quality improvement strategies based on our experiences within the Cochrane Effective Practice and Organisation of Care group. The main limitation of current systematic reviews (and the main challenge confronting reviewers) is the quality of evaluations of quality improvement strategies. Fortunately, well done systematic reviews provide guidance for future studies. Indeed, at present the main contribution of systematic reviews in this area may be to highlight the need for more rigorous evaluations, but there are indications that the quality of evaluations is improving.[20] Those planning and reporting evaluations of quality improvement should do so in the context of a systematic review. Similarly, those planning quality improvement activities should consider the results of systematic reviews when doing so.

Key messages

- Systematic reviews provide the best evidence on the effectiveness of healthcare interventions including quality improvement strategies.
- Systematic reviews allow the generalisability and consistency of research findings to be assessed and data inconsistencies to be explored across studies.
- The conduct of systematic reviews requires content and technical expertise.
- The Cochrane Effective Practice and Organisation of Care (EPOC) group has developed methods and tools to support reviews of quality improvement strategies.

Acknowledgements

The Cochrane Effective Practice and Organisation of Care (EPOC) group is funded by the UK Department of Health. Jeremy Grimshaw holds a Canada Research Chair in Health Knowledge Transfer and Uptake. The Health Services Research Unit is funded by the Chief Scientist Office of the Scottish Office Department of Health. The views expressed are those of the authors and not necessarily of the funding bodies. Phil Alderson became an EPOC editor in September 2002; the development of many of these methods predated his arrival and Phil did not consider his contribution sufficient for authorship. We would like to acknowledge his ongoing contribution to EPOC.

We would like to thank all the reviewers who have undertaken quality improvement reviews and helped us to develop many of the ideas within this chapter. This chapter reflects our experiences of undertaking reviews of quality improvement strategies over the last decade. It promotes some of the tools developed by EPOC over this time period, most of which are available freely from our website. We hope that this chapter will increase the number and quality of systematic reviews of quality improvement strategies and that some of these will be done in collaboration with EPOC.

Potential conflict of interest: The authors are all associated with the Cochrane Effective Practice and Organisation of Care group.

References

1 Cochrane Collaboration. Glossary. *Cochrane Library.* Issue 2. Oxford: Update Software, 2003.
2 NHS Centre for Reviews and Dissemination. *Effect Health Care* 1999;5:1–16.
3 Grimshaw JM, Shirran L, Thomas R, *et al.* Changing provider behavior: an overview of systematic reviews of interventions. *Med Care* 2001;**39**(suppl 2):II2–45.
4 Grimshaw JM, Eccles MP, Walker AE, *et al.* Changing physician behavior. What works and thoughts on getting more things to work. *J Cont Educ Health Professionals* 2002;**22**:237–43.
5 Chalmers I. Trying to do more good than harm in policy and practice: the role of rigorous, transparent, up-to-date, replicable evaluations. *Ann Am Acad Political Soc Sci* 2003 (in press).
6 Mulrow CD. Systematic reviews: rationale for systematic reviews. *BMJ* 1994;**309**:597–9.
7 Mowatt G, Grimshaw JM, Davis D, *et al.* Getting evidence into practice: the work of the Cochrane Effective Practice and Organisation of Care Group (EPOC). *J Cont Educ Health Professions* 2001;**21**:55–60.
8 Alderson P, Bero L, Grilli R, *et al*, eds. Cochrane Effective Professional and Organisation of Care Group. In: *Cochrane Library*. Issue 2. Oxford: Update Software, 2003.
9 Effective Practice and Organisation of Care Group (EPOC). 2003. http://www.epoc.uottawa.ca (accessed 27 April 2003).
10 Clarke M, Oxman AD, eds. Cochrane Reviewers' Handbook 4.1.6. *Cochrane Library*. Issue 2. Oxford: Update Software, 2003. Updated quarterly.
11 Egger M, Davey Smith G, Altman DG, eds. *Systematic reviews in health care. Meta-analysis in context.* London: BMJ Publishing, 2001.
12 Cooper H, Hedges LV, eds. *The handbook of research synthesis*. New York: Russell Sage Foundation, 1994.
13 Egger M, Davey Smith G. Principles and procedures for systematic reviews. In: Egger M, Davey Smith G, Altman DG, eds. *Systematic reviews in health care. Meta-analysis in context.* London: BMJ Publishing, 2001.
14 Eccles M, Grimshaw J, Campbell M, *et al.* Research designs for studies evaluating the effectiveness of change and improvement strategies. *Qual Saf Health Care* 2003;**12**:47–52.

15 Grilli R, Ramsay CR, Minozzi S. Mass media interventions: effects on health services utilisation (Cochrane Review). *Cochrane Library*. Issue 2. Oxford: Update Software, 2003.
16 Effective Practice and Organisation of Care Group (EPOC). *The data collection checklist, section 2.1.1.* http://www.epoc.uottawa.ca/checklist2002.doc (accessed 27 April 2003).
17 Gotzsche PC. Why we need a broad perspective on meta-analysis. *BMJ* 2000;**321**:585–6.
18 Jamtvedt G, Young JM, Kristoffersen DT, *et al*. Audit and feedback: effects on professional practice and health care outcomes (Cochrane Review). *Cochrane Library*. Issue 2. Oxford: Update Software, 2003.
19 Oxman AD, Guyatt GH. A consumer's guide to subgroup analyses. *Ann Intern Med* 1992;**116**:78–84.
20 Lefebvre C, Clarke MJ. Identifying randomised trials. In: Eggar M, Davey Smith G, Altman DG, eds. *Systematic reviews in health care. Meta-analysis in context*. London: BMJ Publishing, 2001.
21 Grimshaw JM, Thomas RE, MacLennan G, *et al*. Effectiveness and efficiency of guideline dissemination and implementation strategies. *Health Technol Assess* 2003 (in press).
22 Juni P, Altman DG, Eggar M. Assessing the quality of randomised controlled trials. In: Eggar M, Davey Smith G, Altman DG, eds. *Systematic reviews in health care. Meta-analysis in context*. London: BMJ Publishing, 2001.
23 Cook TD, Campbell DT. *Quasi-experimentation: design and analysis issues for field settings*. Chicago: Rand McNally, 1979.
24 Whiting-O'Keefe QE, Henke C, Simborg DW. Choosing the correct unit of analysis in medical care experiments. *Med Care* 1984;**22**:1101–14.
25 Ukoumunne OC, Gulliford MC, Chinn S, *et al*. Methods for evaluating area-wide and organisation based interventions in health and health care: a systematic review. *Health Technol Assess* 1999; **3**(5).
26 Rao JNK, Scott AJ. A simple method for the analysis of clustered binary data. *Biometrics* 1992;**48**:577–85.
27 Donner A, Klar N. Issues in meta-analysis of cluster randomised trials. *Stat Med* 2002;**21**:2971–80.
28 Ramsay C, Matowe L, Grilli R, *et al*. Interrupted time series designs in health technology assessment: lessons from two systematic reviews of behaviour change strategies. *Int J Technol Assess Health Care* 2003 (in press).
29 Peto R. Why do we need systematic overviews of randomised trials? *Stat Med* 1987;**6**:233–41.
30 Bushman BJ. Vote counting methods in meta-analysis. In: Cooper H, Hedges L, eds. *The handbook of research synthesis*. New York: Russell Sage Foundation, 1994.
31 Freemantle N, Harvey EL, Wolf F, *et al*. Printed educational materials: effects on professional practice and health care outcomes (Cochrane Review). *Cochrane Library*. Issue 1. Oxford: Update Software, 1997.
32 Thompson SG. Why sources of heterogeneity in meta-analysis should be investigated. *BMJ* 1994;**309**:1351–5.
33 Sterne JAC, Egger M, Davey Smith G. Investigating and dealing with publication and other biases. In: Eggar M, Davey Smith G, Altman DG, eds. *Systematic reviews in health care. Meta-analysis in context*. London: BMJ Publishing, 2001.
34 Oxman AD. Checklists for review articles. *BMJ* 1994;**309**:648–51.
35 Oxman AD, Guyatt GH. The science of reviewing research. *Ann NY Acad Sci* 1993;**703**:123–31.

7: Research designs for studies evaluating the effectiveness of change and improvement strategies

MARTIN ECCLES, JEREMY GRIMSHAW, MARION CAMPBELL, CRAIG RAMSAY

The methods of evaluating change and improvement strategies are not well described. The design and conduct of a range of experimental and non-experimental quantitative designs are considered. Such study designs should usually be used in a context where they build on appropriate theoretical, qualitative, and modelling work, particularly in the development of appropriate interventions. A range of experimental designs are discussed including single and multiple arm randomised controlled trials and the use of more complex factorial and block designs. The impact of randomisation at both group and individual levels and three non-experimental designs (uncontrolled before and after, controlled before and after, and time series analysis) are also considered. The design chosen will reflect both the needs (and resources) in any particular circumstances and also the purpose of the evaluation. The general principle underlying the choice of evaluative design is, however, simple – those conducting such evaluations should use the most robust design possible to minimise bias and maximise generalisability.

There is a substantial literature about the design, conduct, and analysis of evaluations of relatively simple healthcare interventions such as drugs. However, the methods of evaluating complex interventions such as quality improvement interventions are less well described. Evaluation informs the choice between alternative interventions or policies by identifying, estimating, and, if possible, valuing the advantages and disadvantages of each.[1]

Box 7.1 Possible quantitative evaluative designs for quality improvement research

Randomised designs
- Individual patient randomised controlled trials
- Cluster randomised trials

Non-randomised designs
- Uncontrolled before and after studies
- Controlled before and after studies
- Time series designs

There are a number of quantitative designs that could be used to evaluate quality improvement interventions (Box 7.1).

All of these designs attempt to establish general causal relationships across a population of interest. The choice of design will be dependent upon the purpose of the evaluation and the degree of control the researchers have over the delivery of the intervention(s). In general, researchers should choose a design that minimises potential bias (any process at any stage of inference which tends to produce results or conclusions that differ systematically from the truth; also referred to as internal validity) and maximises generalisability (the degree to which the results of a study hold true for situations other than those pertaining to the study, in particular for routine clinical practice; also referred to as external validity).[2,3]

A framework for evaluating quality improvement interventions

Campbell et al[4] have suggested that the evaluation of complex interventions should follow a sequential approach involving:

- development of the theoretical basis for an intervention
- definition of components of the intervention (using modelling, simulation techniques, or qualitative methods)

- exploratory studies to develop further the intervention and plan a definitive evaluative study (using a variety of methods)
- definitive evaluative study (using quantitative evaluative methods, predominantly randomised designs).

This framework demonstrates the interrelation between quantitative evaluative methods and other methods; it also makes explicit that the design and conduct of quantitative evaluative studies should build upon the findings of other quality improvement research. However, it represents an idealised framework and, in some circumstances, it is necessary to undertake evaluations without sequentially working through the earlier stages – for example, when evaluating policy interventions that are being introduced without prior supporting evidence.

In this chapter we describe quantitative approaches for evaluating quality improvement interventions, focusing on methods for estimating the magnitude of the benefits. We also focus on the evaluation of interventions within systems rather than evaluations of whole systems. We discuss several study designs for definitive evaluative studies including a range of randomised controlled trial designs and three non-randomised or quasi-experimental evaluative designs.

Evaluative designs

Randomised designs

Randomised trials are the gold standard method for evaluating healthcare interventions.[5] They estimate the impact of an intervention through direct comparison with a randomly allocated control group that receives either no intervention or an alternative intervention.[6] The randomisation process is the best way of ensuring that both known and (particularly importantly) unknown factors (confounders) that may independently affect the outcome of an intervention are likely to be distributed evenly between the trial groups. As a result, differences observed between groups can be more confidently ascribed to the effects of the intervention rather than to other factors. The same arguments that are used to justify randomised controlled trials of clinical interventions such as drugs are at least as salient to the evaluations of quality improvement interventions. In particular, given our incomplete understanding of potential confounders relating to organisational or professional performance, it is even more difficult to adjust for these in non-randomised designs.

Cluster randomisation

While it is possible to conduct randomised trials of quality improvement interventions which randomise individual patients, this may not always be ideal. If there is the possibility that the treatment given to control individuals will be affected by an organisation's or professional's experience of applying the intervention to other patients in the experimental group, there is a risk of contamination. For example, Morgan et al.[7] investigated the effects of computerised reminders for antenatal care. Patients were randomised and physicians received reminders for intervention patients but not control patients. Compliance in intervention patients rose from 83% to 98% over 6 months, while compliance in control patients rose from 83% to 94% over 12 months. This is a probable contamination effect.

If such contamination is likely, the researcher should consider randomising organisations or healthcare professionals rather than individual patients, although data may still be collected about the process and outcome of care at the individual patient level. Such trials, which randomise at one level (organisation or professional) and collect data at a different level (patient), are known as cluster randomised trials.[8,9] Cluster randomisation has considerable implications for the design, power, and analysis of studies which have frequently been ignored.

Design considerations The main design considerations concern the level of randomisation and whether to include baseline measurement. Frequently researchers need to trade off the likelihood of contamination at lower levels of randomisation against decreasing numbers of clusters and increasing logistical problems at higher levels of randomisation. For example, in a study of an educational intervention in secondary care settings, potential levels of randomisation would include the individual clinician, the ward, the clinical service or directorate, and the hospital. Randomisation at the level of the hospital would minimise the risk of contamination but dramatically increase the size and complexity of the study due to the greater number of hospitals required. Randomisation at the level of the individual clinician would decrease the number of hospitals required but there may then be a risk of contamination across clinicians working in the same wards or specialty areas.

In situations where relatively few clusters (for example, hospitals) are available for randomisation, there is increased danger of imbalance in performance between study and control groups due to the play of chance. Baseline measurements can be used to assess adequacy of the allocation process and are also useful because they provide an estimate of the magnitude of a problem. Low performance scores before the intervention may indicate that performance is poor and there is much room for improvement, whereas high performance scores may indicate that there is little room for improvement (ceiling effect). In addition, baseline measures could be used as a stratifying or matching variable or incorporated in the analysis to increase statistical power (see below). These potential benefits have to be weighed against the increased costs and duration of studies incorporating baseline measurements and concerns about testing effects (introduction of potential bias due to sensitisation of the study subjects during baseline measurement).[2]

Sample size calculation A fundamental assumption of the standard statistics used to analyse patient randomised trials is that the outcome for an individual patient is completely unrelated to that for any other patient – they are said to be "independent". This assumption is violated, however, when cluster randomisation is adopted because two patients within any one cluster are more likely to respond in a similar manner than are two patients from different clusters. For example, the management of patients in a single hospital is more likely to be consistent than management of patients across a number of hospitals. The primary consequence of adopting a cluster randomised design is that it is not as statistically efficient and has lower statistical power than a patient randomised trial of equivalent size.

Sample sizes for cluster randomised trials therefore need to be inflated to adjust for clustering. A statistical measure of the extent of clustering is known as the "intracluster correlation coefficient" (ICC) which is based on the relationship of the between-cluster to within-cluster variance.[10] Table 7.1 shows a number of ICCs from a primary care study of computerising guidelines for patients with either asthma or stable angina (Box 7.4).

Both the ICC and the cluster size influence the inflation required; the sample size inflation can be considerable especially if the average cluster size is large. The extra numbers of patients required can be achieved by increasing either the number of clusters in the study (the more efficient method[11]) or the number of patients per cluster. In general, little additional power is gained from increasing the number of patients per cluster above 50. Researchers often have to trade off the logistical difficulties and costs associated with recruitment of extra clusters against those associated with increasing the number of patients per cluster.[12]

Analysis of cluster randomised trials There are three general approaches to the analysis of cluster randomised trials: analysis at cluster level, the adjustment of standard tests, and advanced statistical techniques using data recorded at both the individual and cluster level.[9,13,14] Cluster level analyses use the cluster as the unit of randomisation and analysis. A summary statistic (for example, mean, proportion) is computed for each cluster and, as each cluster provides only one data point, the data can be considered to be independent, allowing standard statistical tests to be used. Patient level analyses can be undertaken using adjustments to simple statistical tests to account for the clustering effect. However, this approach does not allow adjustment for patient or practice characteristics. Recent advances in the development and use of new modelling techniques to incorporate patient level data allow the inherent correlation within clusters to be modelled explicitly, and thus a "correct" model can be obtained. These methods can incorporate the hierarchical nature of the data into the analysis. For example, in a primary care setting we may have patients (level 1) treated by general practitioners (level 2) nested within practices (level 3) and may

Table 7.1 ICCs for medical record and prescribing data

Angina		**Asthma**	
Process of care measures			
Number of consultations	0·04	Number of consultations	0·03
Number of consultations for angina	0·16	Number of consultations for asthma	0·05
Was blood pressure recorded?	0·04	Compliance checked?	0·15
Was exercise level or advice about exercise recorded?	0·08	Inhaler technique checked?	0·10
		Lung function recorded?	0·08
Any advice about Mediterranean diet or oily fish?	0·01	Asthma education recorded?	0·12
		Smoking status recorded?	0·09
Weight or advice about weight recorded?	0·10	Smoking advice/education recorded?	0·03
Smoking status recorded?	0·10		
ECG recorded?	0·01		
Thyroid function recorded?	0·01		
Blood glucose or HbA1c recorded?	0·03		
Cholesterol or other lipids recorded?	0·04		
Haemoglobin recorded?	0·05		
Exercise ECG recorded?	0·02		
Drugs			
Was verapamil prescribed?	0·01	Was a short acting β2 agonist prescribed?	0·02
Was a beta blocker prescribed?	0·01		
Short acting GTN	0·01	Inhaled corticosteroids	0·02
Modified release GTN	0·01	Long acting β2 agonists	0·01
Transdermal GTN	0·02	Oral steroids	0·02
Isosorbide dinitrate (SA & MR)	0·07	Oral bronchodilators	0·02
Isosorbide mononitrate (SA & MR)	0·02	Prescribing of inhaled corticosteroids for subjects who were prescribed a mean daily dose of > 6 puffs	0·04
Diltiazem	0·02		
Ca channel blocker	0·01		
Statins	0·02		
Beta blocker and dinitrate	0·04		
Calcium blocker and dinitrate	0·04		
Nitrate, calcium blocker and β blocker	0·02		

have covariates measured at the patient level (for example, patient age or sex), the general practitioner level (for example, sex, time in practice), and at the practice level (for example, practice size). Which of the methods is better to use is still a topic of debate. The main advantage of such sophisticated statistical methods is their flexibility. However, they require extensive computing time and statistical expertise, both for the execution of the procedures and in the interpretation of the results.

No consensus exists as to which approach should be used. The most appropriate analysis option will depend on a number of factors including the research question, the unit of inference, the study design, whether the researchers wish to adjust for other relevant variables at the individual or cluster level (covariates), the type and distribution of outcome measure, the number of clusters randomised, the size of cluster and variability of cluster size, and statistical resources available in the research team. Campbell et al[15] and Mollison et al[16] present worked examples comparing these different analytical strategies.

Possible types of cluster randomised trials

Two arm trials The simplest randomised design is the two arm trial where each subject is randomised to study or control groups. Observed differences in performance between the groups are assumed to be due to the intervention. Such trials are relatively straightforward to design and conduct and they maximise statistical power (half the sample is allocated to the intervention and half to the control). However, they only provide information about the effectiveness of a single intervention compared with control (or the relative effectiveness of two interventions without reference to a control). Box 7.2 shows an example of a two arm trial.

Multiple arm trials The simplest extension to the two arm trial is to randomise groups of professionals to more than two groups – for example, two or more study groups and a control group. Such studies are relatively simple to design and use, and allow head to head comparisons of interventions or levels of intervention under similar circumstances. These benefits are, however, compromised by a loss of statistical power; for example, to achieve the same power as a two arm trial, the sample size for a three arm trial needs to be increased by up to 50%.

Factorial designs Factorial designs allow the evaluation of the relative effectiveness of more than one intervention

Box 7.2 Two arm trial[17]

The trial aimed to assess whether the quality of cardiovascular preventive care in general practice could be improved through a comprehensive intervention implemented by an educational outreach visitor. After baseline measurements, 124 general practices (in the southern half of the Netherlands) were randomly allocated to either intervention or control. The intervention, based on the educational outreach model, comprised 15 practice visits over a period of 21 months and addressed a large number of issues around task delegation, availability of instruments and patient leaflets, record keeping, and follow up routines. Twenty one months after the start of the intervention, post-intervention measurements were performed. The difference between ideal and actual practice in each aspect of organising preventive care was defined as a deficiency score. The primary outcome measure was the difference in deficiency scores before and after the intervention. All practices completed both baseline and post-intervention measurements. The difference in change between intervention and control groups, adjusted for baseline, was statistically significant ($p < 0{\cdot}001$) for each aspect of organising preventive care. The largest absolute improvement was found for the number of preventive tasks performed by the practice assistant.

compared with control. For example, in a 2×2 factorial design evaluating two interventions against control, participants are randomised to each intervention (A and B) independently. In the first randomisation the study participants are randomised to intervention A or control. In the second randomisation the same participants are randomised to intervention B or control. This results in four groups: no intervention, intervention A alone, intervention B alone, interventions A and B.

During the analysis of factorial designs it is possible to undertake independent analyses to estimate the effect of the interventions separately[18]; essentially this design allows the conduct of two randomised trials for the same sample size as a two arm trial. However, these trials are more difficult to operationalise and analyse, they provide only limited power for a direct head-to-head comparison of the two interventions, and the power is diminished if there is interaction between the two interventions. Box 7.3 shows an example of a factorial design trial that was powered to be able to detect any interaction effects.

Box 7.3 Factorial design[19]

The trial evaluated the effectiveness of audit and feedback and educational reminder messages in changing general practitioners' radiology ordering behaviour for lumber spine and knee *x* rays. The design was a before and after pragmatic cluster randomised controlled trial using a 2 × 2 factorial design involving 244 practices and six radiology departments in two geographical regions. Each practice was randomised twice, to receive or not each of the two interventions. Educational reminder messages were based on national guidelines and were provided on the report of every relevant *x* ray ordered during the 12 month intervention period. For example, the lumbar spine message read "In either acute (less than 6 weeks) or chronic back pain, without adverse features, *x* ray is not routinely indicated". The audit and feedback covered the preceding 6 month period and was delivered to individual general practitioners at the start of the intervention period and again 6 months later. It provided practice level information relating the number of requests made by the whole practice relative to the number of requests made by all practices in the study. Audit and feedback led to a non-significant relative reduction of around 1% *x* ray requests while educational reminder messages led to a significant reduction of about 20%.

Balanced incomplete block designs In guideline implementation research there are a number of non-specific effects which may influence the estimate of the effect of an intervention. These could be positive attention effects from participants knowing that they are the subject of a study, or negative demotivation effects from being allocated to a control rather than an intervention group. Currently, these non-specific effects are grouped together and termed the "Hawthorne effect". If these are not balanced across study groups in a quality improvement trial, the resulting estimates of effects may be biased and, as these effects can potentially be of the same order of magnitude as the effects that studies are seeking to demonstrate, there is an advantage to dealing with them systematically. While these effects may be difficult to eliminate, balanced incomplete block designs can be used to equalise such non-specific effects and thereby minimise their impact.[18] An example is shown in Box 7.4.

Box 7.4 Balanced incomplete block design[20]

This study was a before and after pragmatic cluster randomised controlled trial using a 2 × 2 incomplete block design and was designed to evaluate the use of a computerised decision support system (CDSS) in implementing evidence-based clinical guidelines for the primary care management of angina and asthma in adults. It was based in 60 general practices in the north east of England and the participants were general practitioners and practice nurses in the study practices and their patients aged 18 years or over and with angina or asthma. The practices were randomly allocated to two groups. The first group received computerised guidelines for the management of angina and provided intervention patients for the management of angina and control patients for the management of asthma. The second received computerised guidelines for the management of asthma and provided intervention patients for the management of asthma and control patients for the management of angina. The outcome measures were adherence to the guidelines, determined by recording of care in routine clinical records, and any subsequent impact measured by patient reported generic and condition specific measures of outcome. There were no significant effects of CDSS on consultation rates, process of care measures (including prescribing), or any quality of life domain for either condition. Levels of use of the CDSS were low.

As doctors in both groups were subject to the same level of intervention, any non-specific effects are equalised across the two groups leaving any resulting difference as being due to the intervention.

Non-randomised designs

Quasi-experimental designs

Quasi-experimental designs are useful where there are political, practical, or ethical barriers to conducting a genuine (randomised) experiment. Under such circumstances, researchers have little control over the delivery of an intervention and have to plan an evaluation around a proposed intervention. A large number of potential designs have been summarised by Campbell and Stanley,[2] and Cook and Campbell.[3] Here we discuss the three most commonly used designs in quality improvement studies: (1) uncontrolled before and after studies, (2) controlled before and after studies, and (3) time series designs.

Uncontrolled before and after studies Uncontrolled before and after studies measure performance before and after the introduction of an intervention in the same study site(s) and observed differences in performance are assumed to be due to the intervention. They are relatively simple to conduct and are superior to observational studies, but they are intrinsically weak evaluative designs because secular trends or sudden changes make it difficult to attribute observed changes to the intervention. There is some evidence to suggest that the results of uncontrolled before and after studies may overestimate the effects of quality improvement-like interventions. Lipsey and Wilson[21] undertook an overview of meta-analyses of psychological, educational, and behavioural interventions. They identified 45 reviews that reported separately the pooled estimates from controlled and uncontrolled studies, and noted that the observed effects from uncontrolled studies were greater than those from controlled studies. In general, uncontrolled before and after studies should not be used to evaluate the effects of quality improvement interventions and the results of studies using such designs have to be interpreted with great caution.

Controlled before and after studies In controlled before and after studies the researcher attempts to identify a control population of similar characteristics and performance to the study population and collects data in both populations before and after the intervention is applied to the study population. Analysis compares post-intervention performance or change scores in the study and control groups and observed differences are assumed to be due to the intervention.

While well designed before and after studies should protect against secular trends and sudden changes, it is often difficult to identify a comparable control group. Even in apparently well matched control and study groups, performance at baseline often differs. Under these circumstances, "within group" analyses are often undertaken (where change from baseline is compared within both groups separately and where the assumption is made that, if the change in the intervention group is significant and the change in the control group is not, the intervention has had an effect). Such analyses are inappropriate for a number of reasons. Firstly, the baseline imbalance suggests that the control group is not truly comparable and may not experience the same secular trends or sudden changes as the intervention group; thus any apparent effect of the intervention may be spurious. Secondly, there is no direct comparison between study and control groups.[2] Another common analytical problem in practice is that researchers fail to recognise clustering of data when interventions are delivered at an organisational level and data are collected at the individual patient level.

Time series designs Time series designs attempt to detect whether an intervention has had an effect significantly greater than the underlying secular trend.[3] They are useful in quality improvement research for evaluating the effects of interventions when it is difficult to randomise or identify an appropriate control group – for example, following the dissemination of national guidelines or mass media campaigns (Box 7.5). Data are collected at multiple time points before and after the intervention. The multiple time points before the intervention allow the underlying trend and any cyclical (seasonal) effects to be estimated, and the multiple time points after the intervention allow the intervention effect to be estimated while taking account of the underlying secular trends.

Box 7.5 Time series analysis[22]

An interrupted time series using monthly data for 34 months before and 14 months after dissemination of the guidelines was used to evaluate the effect of postal dissemination of the third edition of the Royal College of Radiologists' guidelines on general practitioner referrals for radiography. Data were abstracted for the period April 1994 to March 1998 from the computerised administrative systems of open access radiological services provided by two teaching hospitals in one region of Scotland. A total of 117 747 imaging requests from general practice were made during the study period. There were no significant effects of disseminating the guidelines on the total number of requests or 18 individual tests. If a simple before and after design was used, then the authors would have erroneously concluded that 11 of the 18 procedures had significant differences.

The most important influence on the analysis technique is the number of data points collected before the intervention. It is necessary to collect enough data points to be convinced that a stable estimate of the underlying secular trend has been obtained. There are a number of statistical techniques that can be used depending on the characteristics of the data, the number of data points available, and whether autocorrelation is present.[3] Autocorrelation refers to the situation where data points collected close in time are likely to be more similar to each other than data points collected far apart. For example, for any given month the waiting times in hospitals are likely to be more similar to waiting times in adjacent months than to waiting times 12 months previously. Autocorrelation has to be allowed for in analysis and time series regression models,[23] and autoregressive integrated moving averages (ARIMA) modelling[3] and time series regression models[23] are all methods for dealing with this problem.

Well designed time series evaluations increase the confidence with which the estimate of effect can be attributed to the intervention, although the design does not provide protection against the effects of other events occurring at the same time as the study intervention which might also improve performance. Furthermore, it is often difficult to collect sufficient data points unless routine data sources are available. It has been found that many published time series studies have been inappropriately analysed, frequently resulting in an overestimation of the effect of the intervention.[24,25]

Discussion

Randomised trials should only be considered when there is genuine uncertainty about the effectiveness of an intervention. Whilst they are the optimal design for evaluating quality improvement interventions, they are not without their problems. They can be logistically difficult, especially if the researchers are using complex designs to evaluate more than one intervention or if cluster randomisation – requiring the recruitment of large numbers of clusters – is planned. They are undoubtedly methodologically challenging and require a multidisciplinary approach to adequately plan and conduct. They can also be time consuming and expensive; in our experience a randomised trial of a quality improvement intervention can rarely be completed in less than two years.

Critics of randomised trials frequently express concerns that tight inclusion criteria of trials or artificial constraints placed upon participants limit the generalisability of the findings. While this is a particular concern in efficacy (explanatory) studies of drugs, it is likely to be less of a problem in quality improvement evaluations that are likely to be inherently pragmatic.[26] Pragmatic studies aim to test whether an intervention is likely to be effective in routine practice by comparing the new procedure against the current regimen; as such they are the most useful trial design for developing policy recommendations. Such studies attempt to approximate normal conditions and do not attempt to equalise contextual factors and other effect modifiers in the intervention and study groups. In pragmatic studies, the contextual and effect modifying factors therefore become part of the interventions. Such studies are usually conducted on a predefined study population and withdrawals are included within an "intention to treat" analysis: all subjects initially allocated to the intervention group would be analysed as intervention subjects irrespective of whether they received the intervention or not. For example, in an evaluation of a computerised decision support system as a method of delivering clinical guidelines in general practice (Box 7.4), some general practitioners may not have had the computing skills to work the intervention. In an intention to treat analysis, data from all general practitioners would be included in the analysis irrespective of whether they could use the system or not; as a result, the estimates of effect would more likely reflect the effectiveness of the intervention in real world settings.

The main limitation of quasi-experimental designs is that the lack of randomised controls threatens internal validity and increases the likelihood of plausible rival hypotheses. Shadish et al[3] provide a framework for considering the internal validity of the results of experiments and quasi-experiments when trying to establish causality. They suggest that "the task of individually assessing the plausibility of internal validity threats is definitely more laborious and less certain than relying on experimental design, randomisation in particular." Within quasi-experiments there are potentially greater threats to internal validity and less ability to account for these. We believe that the design and conduct of quasi-experimental studies is at least as methodologically challenging as the design and conduct of randomised trials. The generalisability of quasi-experimental designs is also uncertain. Many quasi-experimental studies are conducted in a small number of study sites which may not be representative of the population to which the researcher wishes to generalise.

Conclusions

We have considered a range of research designs for studies evaluating the effectiveness of change and improvement strategies. The design chosen will reflect both the needs (and resources) in any particular circumstances and also the purpose of the evaluation. The general principle underlying the choice of evaluative design is, however, simple – those conducting such evaluations should use the most robust design possible to minimise bias and maximise generalisability.

Key messages

- Whatever design is chosen, it is important to minimise bias and maximise generalisability.
- Quantitative designs should be used within a sequence of evaluation, building as appropriate on preceding theoretical, qualitative, and modelling work.
- There are a range of more or less complex randomised designs.
- When using randomised designs it is important to consider the appropriate use of cluster, rather than individual, randomisation. This has implications for both study design and analysis.
- Where randomised designs are not feasible, non-randomised designs can be used although they are more susceptible to bias.

Acknowledgements

The Health Services Research Unit is funded by the Chief Scientist Office, Scottish Executive Department of Health. The views expressed are those of the authors and not the funding bodies. Jeremy Grimshaw holds a Canada Research Chair in Health Knowledge Transfer and Uptake.

References

1 Russell IT. The evaluation of a computerised tomography: a review of research methods. In: Culyer AJ, Horisberger B, eds. *Economic and medical evaluation of health care technologies*. Berlin: Springer-Verlag, 1983: 38–68.
2 Campbell DT, Stanley J. *Experimental and quasi-experimental designs for research*. Chicago: Rand McNally, 1966.
3 Shadish WR, Cook TD, Campbell DT. *Experimental and quasi-experimental designs for generalized causal inference*. Boston: Houghton Mifflin, 2002.
4 Campbell M, Fitzpatrick R, Haines A, *et al*. Framework for design and evaluation of complex interventions to improve health. *BMJ* 2000;**321**: 694–6.
5 Cochrane AL. *Effectiveness and efficiency: random reflections on health services*. London: Nuffield Provincial Hospitals Trust, 1979.
6 Pocock SJ. *Clinical trials: a practical approach*. New York: Wiley, 1983.
7 Morgan M, Studney DR, Barnett GO, *et al*. Computerized concurrent review of prenatal care. *Qual Rev Bull* 1978;**4**:33–6.
8 Donner A, Klar N. *Design and analysis of cluster randomization trials in health research*. London: Arnold, 2000.
9 Murray DM. *The design and analysis of group randomised trials*. Oxford: Oxford University Press, 1998.
10 Donner A, Koval JJ. The estimation of intraclass correlation in the analysis of family data. *Biometrics* 1980;**36**:19–25.
11 Diwan VK, Eriksson B, Sterky G, *et al*. Randomization by group in studying the effect of drug information in primary care. *Int J Epidemiol* 1992;**21**:124–30.
12 Flynn TN, Whitley E, Peters TJ. Recruitment strategies in a cluster randomised trial – cost implications. *Stat Med* 2002;**21**:397–405.
13 Donner A. Some aspects of the design and analysis of cluster randomization trials. *Appl Stat* 1998;**47**:95–113.
14 Turner MJ, Flannelly GM, Wingfield M, *et al*. The miscarriage clinic: an audit of the first year. *Br J Obstet Gynaecol* 1991;**98**:306–8.
15 Campbell MK, Mollison J, Steen N, *et al*. Analysis of cluster randomized trails in primary care: a practical approach. *Fam Pract* 2000;**17**: 192–6.
16 Mollison JA, Simpson JA, Campbell MK, *et al*. Comparison of analytical methods for cluster randomised trials: an example from a primary care setting. *J Epidemiol Biostat* 2000;**5**:339–48.
17 Lobo CM, Frijling BD, Hulscher MEJL, *et al*. Improving quality of organising cardiovascular preventive care in general practice by outreach visitors: a randomised controlled trial. *Prev Med* 2002;**35**:422–9.
18 Cochran WG, Cox GM. *Experimental design*. New York: Wiley, 1957.
19 Eccles M, Steen N, Grimshaw J, *et al*. Effect of audit and feedback, and reminder messages on primary-care radiology referrals: a randomised trial. *Lancet* 2001;**357**:1406–9.
20 Eccles M, McColl E, Steen N, *et al*. A cluster randomised controlled trial of computerised evidence based guidelines for angina and asthma in primary care. *BMJ* 2002;**325**:941–7.
21 Lipsey MW, Wilson DB. The efficacy of psychological, educational, and behavioral treatment: confirmation from meta-analysis. *Am Psychol* 1993;**48**:1181–209.
22 Matowe L, Ramsay C, Grimshaw JM, *et al*. Influence of the Royal College of Radiologists' guidelines on referrals from general practice: a time series analysis. *Clin Radiol* 2002;**57**:575–8.

23 Ostrom CW. *Time series analysis: regression techniques*. London: Sage, 1990.
24 Grilli R, Ramsay CR, Minozzi S. Mass media interventions: effects on health services utilisation (Cochrane Review). *Cochrane Library.* Oxford: Update Software, 2002.
25 Grilli R, Freemantle N, Minozzi S, *et al.* Impact of mass media on health services utilisation (Cochrane Review). *Cochrane Library*. Issue 3. Oxford: Update Software, 1998.
26 Schwartz D, Lellouch J. Explanatory and pragmatic attitudes in clinical trials. *J Chron Dis* 1967;**20**:648.

8: Evaluation of quality improvement programmes

JOHN ØVRETVEIT, DAVID GUSTAFSON

In response to increasing concerns about quality, many countries are carrying out large scale programmes which include national quality strategies, hospital programmes, and quality accreditation, assessment and review processes. Increasing amounts of resources are being devoted to these interventions, but do they ensure or improve quality of care? There is little research evidence as to their effectiveness or the conditions for maximum effectiveness. Reasons for the lack of evaluation research include the methodological challenges of measuring outcomes and attributing causality to these complex, changing, long term social interventions in organisations or health systems which themselves are complex and changing. However, methods are available which can be used to evaluate these programmes and which can provide decision makers with research based guidance on how to plan and implement them. This chapter describes the research challenges and the methods which can be used, and gives examples and guidance for future research. It emphasises the important contribution which such research can make to improving the effectiveness of these programmes and to developing the science of quality improvement.

A quality programme is the planned activities carried out by an organisation or health system to improve quality. It covers a range of interventions which are more complex than a single quality team improvement project or the quality activities in one department. Quality programmes include programmes for a whole organisation (such as a hospital total quality programme), for teams from many organisations (for example, a "collaborative" programme), for external reviews of organisations in an area (for example, a quality accreditation programme), for changing practice in many organisations (for example, a practice guidelines formulation and implementation programme), and for a national or regional quality strategy which itself could include any or all of the above. These programmes create conditions which help or hinder smaller quality improvement projects.

Quality improvement programmes are new "social medical technologies" which are increasingly being applied. One study noted 11 different types of programmes in the UK NHS in a recent three year period.[1] They probably consume more resources than any treatment and have potentially greater consequences for patient safety and other clinical outcomes. Yet we know little of their effectiveness or relative cost effectiveness, or how to ensure they are well implemented.

Decision makers and theorists have many questions about these programmes.

- Do they achieve their objectives and, if so, at what cost?
- Why are some more successful than others?
- What are the factors and conditions critical for success?
- What does research tell us about how to improve their effectiveness?

Some anecdotal answers come from the reports of consultants and participants, and there are theories about "critical success factors" for some types of programme. However, until recently there was little independent and systematic research about effectiveness and the conditions for effectiveness. Indeed, there was little descriptive research which documented the activities which people actually undertook when implementing a programme.

Research has made some progress in answering these questions, but perhaps not as much as was hoped, in part because of the methodological challenges. This paper first briefly notes some of the research before describing the challenges and the research designs which can be used. It finishes with suggestions for developing research in this field.

Research into quality improvement programmes

The most studied subcategory of quality programmes is hospital quality programmes, particularly US hospital total quality management programmes (TQM), later called

Box 8.1 Non-systematic reviews of hospital quality programmes

The general conclusions of non-systematic reviews of hospital quality programmes are:

- The label given to a programme (for example, "TQM") is no guide to the activities which are actually carried out: programmes with the same name are implemented very differently at different rates, coverage, and depth in the organisation.
- Few hospitals seem to have achieved significant results and little is known about any long term results.
- Few studies describe or compare different types of hospital quality programmes, especially non-TQM/CQI programmes.
- Most studies have severe limitations (see later).

continuous quality improvement programmes (CQI). Several non-systematic reviews have been carried out (Box 8.1).[2–6]

There is evidence from some studies that certain factors appear to be necessary to motivate and sustain implementation and to create conditions likely to produce results. The most commonly reported are senior management commitment, sustained attention and the right type of management roles at different levels, a focus on customer needs, physician involvement, sufficient resources, careful programme management, practical and relevant training which personnel can use immediately, and the right culture.[4–13] These demanding conditions for success raise questions about whether the type of quality programmes which have been tried are feasible for health care. These limited conclusions appear similar across public and private, and across nations. However, there is little research for non-US clinics and hospitals, for public hospitals, or systematic comparative investigation to support this impression.

With regard to research methods, studies have tended to rely on quality specialists or senior managers for information about the programme and its impact, and to survey them once retrospectively. Future studies need to gather data from a wider range of sources and over a longer period of time. Data should also be gathered to assess the degree of implementation of the programme. Implementation should not be assumed: evidence is needed as to exactly which changes have been made and when. Outcomes need to be viewed in relation to how deeply and broadly the programme was implemented and the stage or "maturity" of the programme. To date, for most studies the lack of evidence of impact may simply reflect the fact that the programmes were not implemented, even though some respondents may say they had been. Assessing the degree of implementation could also help to formulate explanations of outcomes. There is a need for studies of organisations which are similar apart from their use of quality methods and ideas, as well as a need for more studies to use the same measures – for example, of results, of culture, or of other variables. Many of these points also apply to research into other types of quality programmes.

Other quality improvement programmes

Few other types of quality improvement programmes have been systematically studied or evaluated; there are few studies of national or regional programmes such as guideline implementation or of the effectiveness of quality review or accreditation processes.[14] Managers have reported that organisations which received low scores ("probation") on the US Joint Commission on Accreditation of Healthcare Organizations assessment were given high scores three years later but had not made substantive changes.[6] Few studies have described or assessed the validity or value of the many comparative quality assessment systems[15–18] or of external evaluation processes,[19–24] or have studied national or regional quality strategies or programmes in primary health care.[25]

More evaluation research is also being undertaken into quality improvement collaboratives. This is part of a new wave of research which is revealing more about the conditions which organisations and managers need to create in order to foster, sustain, and spread effective projects and changes. Collaboratives are similar to hospital quality programmes in that they usually involve project teams, but the teams are from different organisations. The structure of the collaborative and the steps to be taken are more prescribed than in most hospital quality programmes.

One study has drawn together the results of evaluations of different collaboratives.[26] This study provides knowledge which can be used to develop collaboratives working on other subjects, helps to understand factors critical to success, and also demonstrates other research methods which can be used to study some types of quality programmes. The study concluded that there was some evidence that quality collaboratives can help some teams to make significant improvements quickly if the collaborative is carefully planned and managed, and if the team has the right conditions. It suggested that a team's success depended on their ability to work as a team, their ability to learn and apply quality methods, the strategic importance of their work to their home organisation, the culture of their home organisation, and the type and degree of support from management. This can help teams and their managers to decide whether they have, or can create, the conditions to be able to benefit from taking part in what can be a costly programme.

There is therefore little research into quality programmes which meets rigorous scientific criteria, but some of the research which has been done does provide guidance for decision makers which is more valid than the reports of consultants or participants. There is clearly a need for more evaluations and other types of studies of quality programmes which answer the questions of decision makers and also build theory about large scale interventions to complex health organisations or health systems. The second part of this chapter considers the designs and methods which could be used in future research.

Research challenges

These interventions are difficult to evaluate using experimental methods. Many programmes are evolving, and involve a number of activities which start and finish at different times. These activities may be mutually reinforcing and have a synergistic effect if they are properly implemented: many quality programmes are a "system" of activities. Some quality programmes are implemented over a long period of time; many cannot be standardised and need to be changed to suit the situation in ways which are different from the way in which a treatment is changed to suit a patient.

The targets of the interventions are not patients but whole organisations or social groups which vary more than the physiology of an individual patient: they can be considered as complex adaptive social systems.[27] There are many short and long term outcomes which usually need to be studied from the perspectives of different parties. It is difficult to prove that these outcomes are due to the programme and not to something else, given the changing nature of each type of programme, their target, the environment, and the time scales involved. They are carried out over time in a changing economic, social, and political climate which influences how they are implemented.[28]

One view is that each programme and situation is unique and no generalisations can be made to other programmes elsewhere. This may be true for some programmes, but even then a description of the programme and its context allows others to assess the relevance of the programme and the findings to their local situation. However, at present researchers do not have agreed frameworks to structure their descriptions and allow comparisons, although theories do exist about which factors are critical.

Quasi-experimental designs can be used[29,30]: it may be possible to standardise the intervention, control its implementation, and use comparison programmes within the same environment in order to exclude other possible influences on outcomes. One issue is that many programmes are local interpretations of principles; many are not standardised specific interventions that can be replicated. Indeed, they should not be: flexible implementation for the local situation appears to be important for success.[5] TQM/CQI is more a philosophy and set of principles than a specific set of steps and actions to be implemented by all organisations, although some models do come close to prescribing detailed steps.

Research designs

The difficulties in evaluating these programmes do not mean that they cannot or should not be evaluated. There are a number of designs and methods which can and have been used: these are summarised below and discussed in detail elsewhere.[28–34]

Descriptive case design

This design simply aims to describe the programme as implemented. There is no attempt to gather data about outcomes, but knowledgeable stakeholders' expectations of outcome and perceptions of the strengths and weaknesses of the programme can be gathered. Why is this descriptive design sometimes useful? Some quality programmes are prescribed and standardised – for example, a quality accreditation or external review. In these cases a description of the intervention activities is available which others can use to understand what was done and to replicate the intervention. However, many programmes are implemented in different ways or not described, or may only be described as principles and without a strategy. For the researcher a first description of the programme as implemented saves wasting time looking for impact further down the causal chain (for example, patient outcomes) when few or no activities have actually been implemented.

Audit design

This design takes a written statement about what people should do, such as a protocol or plan, and compares this with what they actually do. This is a quick and low cost evaluation design which is useful when there is evidence that following a programme or protocol will result in certain outcomes. It can be used to describe how far managers and health personnel follow prescriptions for quality programme interventions and why they may diverge from these prescriptions. "Audit" research of quality accreditation or review processes can help managers to develop more cost effective reviews.[35]

Prospective before–after designs: single case or comparative

The single case prospective design gathers specific data about the target of the intervention before and after (or during) the intervention. Outcomes are considered as the differences between the before and after data collected about the target. The immediate target is the organisation and personnel; the ultimate targets are patients.

Comparative before–after designs produce stronger evidence that any outcomes were due to the programme and not to something else. If the comparable unit has no intervention, this design allows some control for competing explanations of outcomes if the units have similar characteristics and environments. These are quasi-experimental or "theory

Box 8.2 A qualitative evaluation of external reviews of clinical governance

One example which illustrates the use of qualitative methods is a study of the UK government's programme of external review of clinical governance arrangements in public healthcare provider organisations.[35] Members of the review team as well as senior clinicians and managers were interviewed in 47 organisations before and after the review. A qualitative analysis identified themes and issues and reported common views about how the review process could be improved.

Although most interviewees thought the reviews gave a valid picture of clinical governance, much of the knowledge produced was already known to them but had not been made explicit. It concluded that major changes in policy, strategy, or direction in the organisations had not occurred as a result of the reviews, and suggested that the use of the same process for all organisations was "at best wasteful of resources and perhaps even positively harmful". This study provided the only independent description of the review process and of different stakeholders' assessments as to its value and how the process could be improved. The findings were useful to the reviewers to refine their programme. One of the limitations of the study was that it did not investigate outcomes further than the interviewees' perceptions of impact: "measuring impact reliably is difficult and different stakeholders may have quite different subjective perceptions of impact".[35]

testing" designs because the researcher predicts changes to the one or more before–after variables, and then gathers the data before and after the intervention (for example, personnel attitudes towards quality) to test the prediction. However, when limited to studying only before–after (or later) differences, these designs do not generate explanations about why any changes occurred (Box 8.2).

Retrospective or concurrent evaluation designs: single case or comparative

In these designs the researcher can use either a quasi-experimental "theory testing" approach or a "theory building" approach. An example of the former is the "prediction testing survey" design. The researcher studies previous theories or empirical research to identify theorised critical success factors – for example, sufficient resources, continuity of

Box 8.3 Example of a theory testing comparative design

The first comprehensive studies of effectiveness of TQM/CQI programmes in health care also tried to establish which factors were critical for "success".[8–10] The methods used in these studies were to survey 67 hospitals, some with programmes and some without, and later 61 hospitals with TQM programmes, asking questions about the programme and relating certain factors to quality performance improvement. The findings were that, after three years, the hospitals could not report clear evidence of results and few had tackled clinical care processes.

A later study tested hypotheses about associations between organisation and cultural factors and performance.[11] Interviews and surveys were undertaken in 10 selected hospitals. Performance improvements were found in most programmes in satisfaction, market share, and economic efficiency as measured by length of stay, unit costs, and labour productivity. Interestingly, culture was only found to influence the patient satisfaction performance. It was easier for smaller hospitals with fewer complex services to implement CQI. Early physician involvement was also associated with CQI success, a finding reported in other studies.[6,7]

This set of studies has a practical value. The findings give managers a reliable foundation for assessing whether they have the conditions which are likely to result in a successful programme. Another strength of this study was to assess the "depth" of implementation by using Baldridge or EFQM award categories.[19,21] Limitations of the study were that precise descriptions of the nature of the different hospital programmes were not given; only one site data gathering visit was undertaken; and less than two years was taken for the investigation so that the way the programmes changed and whether they were sustained could not be gauged. Follow up studies would add to our knowledge of the long term evolution of these programmes, any long term results, and explanations about why some hospitals were more successful than others.

management, aspects of culture – and then tests these to find which are associated with successful and unsuccessful programmes (Box 8.3).

In contrast, a "theory building" approach involves the researcher in gathering data about the intervention, context, and possible effects during or after the intervention (Box 7.4). To describe the programme as it was implemented, the researcher asks different informants to describe the activities which were actually undertaken.[30] The validity of these subjective perceptions can be increased by interviewing a cross

Box 8.4 Example of an action evaluation comparative design

A four year comparative action evaluation study of six Norwegian hospitals provided evidence about results and critical factors.[4,7,36] It gave the first detailed and long term description about what hospitals in a public system actually did and how the programmes changed over time. The study found consistencies between the six sites in the factors critical for success: management and physician involvement at all levels, good data systems, the right training, and effective project team management. A nine year follow up is planned.

section of informants, by asking informants for any evidence which they can suggest which would prove or disprove their perceptions, and by comparing data from difference sources to identify patterns in the data (Box 8.4).[30,32,33]

The choice of design depends on the type of quality programme (short or long term, prescribed or flexible, stable or changing), for whom the research is being undertaken, and the questions to be addressed (Was it carried out as planned? Did it achieve its objectives? What were the outcomes? What explains outcomes or success or failure?). Descriptive, audit, and single case retrospective designs are quicker to complete and are cheaper but do not give information about outcomes. Comparative outcome designs can introduce some degree of control, thus making possible inferences about critical factors if good descriptions of the programmes and their context are also provided.

Improving future research

Some of the shortcomings of research into quality programmes have been presented earlier. The five most common are:

- Implementation assessment failure: the study does not examine the extent to which the programme was actually carried out. Was the intervention implemented fully, in all areas and to the required "depth", and for how long?
- Outcome assessment failure: the study does not assess any outcomes or a sufficiently wide range of outcomes such as

short and long term impact on the organisation, on patients, and on resources consumed.

- Outcome attribution failure: the study does not establish whether the outcomes can unambiguously be attributed to the intervention, or whether something else caused the outcomes.
- Explanation failure: there is no theory or model which explains how the intervention caused the outcomes and which factors and conditions were critical.
- Measurement variability: different researchers use very different data to describe or measure the quality programme process, structure, and outcome. It is therefore difficult to use the results of one study to question or support another or to build up knowledge systematically.

Future evaluations would be improved by attention to the following:

- assessing or measuring the level of implementation of the intervention
- validating "implementation assessment"
- wider outcome assessment
- longitudinal studies
- more attention to economics
- explanatory theory
- common definitions and measures
- tools to predict and explain programme effectiveness.

Assessing or measuring the level of implementation of the intervention

Studies need to assess how "broadly" the programme penetrated the organisation (did it reach all parts?), how "deeply" it was applied in each part, and for how long it was applied. One of the first rules of evaluation is "assume nothing has been implemented – get evidence of what has been implemented, where and for how long".[30] There is no point looking for outcomes until this has been established. Instruments for assessing "stage of implementation" or "maturation" need to be developed such as the adaptation of the Baldridge criteria used in the study by Shortell et al[5] or other instruments (see Chapter 11).

Validating "implementation assessment"

Survey responses are one data source for assessing level of implementation and are useful for selecting organisations for further studies. However, these responses need to be gathered from a cross section of personnel, at different times, and supplemented by site visits and other data sources to improve validity.

Wider outcome assessment

With regard to short term impact, data need to be gathered from a wide cross section of organisational personnel and other stakeholders and from other data sources. Most studies also need to gather data about long term outcomes and to assess carefully the extent to which these outcomes can be attributed to the programme. The outcome data to be gathered should be determined by a theory predicting effects, which builds on previous research, or in terms of the specified objectives of the programme, and these links should be made clear in the report.

Longitudinal studies

Retrospective single surveys provide data which is of limited use. We need more prospective studies which follow the dynamics of the programme over long timescales. Many future studies will need to investigate both the intervention and the outcomes over an extended period of time. Very little is known about whether these programmes are continued and how they might change, or about long term outcomes.

More attention to economics

No studies have assessed the resources consumed by a quality improvement programme or the resource consequences of the outcomes. The suspected high initial costs of implementation would look different if more was known about the costs of sustaining the programme and about the possible savings and economic benefits.[37] Long term evaluations may also uncover more outcomes, benefits, or "side effects" which are not discovered in short studies.

Explanatory theory

For hospital programmes there is no shortage of theories about how to implement them and the conditions needed for success, but few are empirically based. For both practical and scientific reasons, future studies need to test these theories or build theories about what helps and hinders implementation at different stages, and about how the intervention produces any discovered outcomes. For other types of quality programmes there is very little theory of any type. Innovation adoption[38] and diffusion theories are one source of ideas for building explanatory theories, for understanding level of implementation, and for understanding why some organisations are able to apply or benefit more from the intervention than others.[38]

Common definitions and measures

Most studies to date have used their own definitions and measures of effects of quality programmes. This is now limiting our ability to compare and contrast results from different evaluation studies and to build a body of knowledge.

Tools to predict and explain programme effectiveness

Future research needs to go beyond measuring effectiveness and to give decision makers tools to predict the effects of their programmes. Decision theory models could be used to create such tools, as could tools which effectively predict the outcomes of particular improvement projects.[39]

In addition there is a need for overviews and theories of quality improvement programmes; we have not described the full range of interventions which fall within this category and have only given a limited discussion of a few. Future research studies need to describe the range of complex large scale quality interventions increasingly being carried out and their characteristics – for example, to describe and compare national or regional quality programmes. More consideration is needed of the similarities and differences between them, of what can be learned from considering the group as a whole, and of how theories from organisation, change management,

Box 8.5 Steps for studying a quality improvement programme

The methods used depend on who the research is for (the research user), the questions to be addressed, and the type of programme. An example of one action evaluation research strategy is presented here.[30,36]

- Conceptualise the intervention. At an early stage, form a simple model of the component parts of the programme and of the activities carried out at different times. This model can be built up from programme documents or any plans or descriptions which already exist, or from previous theories about the intervention.
- Find and review previous research about similar programmes and make predictions. Identify which factors are suggested by theory or evidence to be critical for the success of the programme. Identify which variables have been studied before and how data were collected.
- Identify research questions which arise out of previous research and/or which are of interest to the users of the research.
- Consider whether the intervention can be controlled in its implementation (would people agree to follow a prescribed approach or have they done so if it is a retrospective study?). If not, design part of the study to gather data to describe the programme as implemented and to assess the level of implementation. Consider whether comparisons could be made with similar or non-intervention sites – for example, to help exclude competing explanations for outcomes or to discover assisting and hindering factors.
- Plan methods to use to investigate how the programme was actually carried out, the different activities performed, and to assess the level of implementation. Gather data about the sequence of activities and how the programme changed over time. Use documentary data sources, observation, interviews, or surveys as appropriate describing how informants or other data sources were selected and possible bias. Note differences between the planned programme and the programme in action, and participants' explanations for this as well as other explanations.
- Plan methods to gather data about the effects of the programme on providers and patients if possible. Data may be participants' subjective perceptions, or more objective before and after data (for example, complaints, clinical outcomes), or both. Use data collected by the programme participants to monitor progress and results if these data are valid. Consider how to capture data about unintended side effects – for example, better personnel recruitment and retention.

(Continued)

Box 8.5 *(Continued)*

- Consider other explanations for discovered effects apart from the programme and assess their plausibility.
- To communicate the findings, create a model of the programme which shows the component parts over time, the main outcomes, and factors and conditions which appear to be critical in producing the outcomes. Specify the limitations of the study, the degree of certainty about the findings, and the answers to the research questions.

sociology, and innovation studies can contribute to building theories about these interventions (Box 8.5).

Conclusions

Although there is research evidence that some discrete quality team projects are effective, there is little evidence that any large scale quality programmes bring significant benefits or are worth the cost. However, neither is there strong evidence that there are no benefits or that resources are being wasted. The changing and complex features of quality programmes, their targets, and the contexts make them difficult to evaluate using conventional medical research experimental evaluation methods, but this does not mean that they cannot be evaluated or investigated in other ways. Quasi-experimental evaluation methods and other social science methods can be used. These methods may not produce the degree of certainty that is produced by a triple blind randomised controlled trial of a treatment, but they can give insights into how these processes work to produce their effects.

Conclusive evidence of effectiveness may never be possible. At this stage a more realistic and useful research strategy is to describe a programme and its context and discover factors which are critical for successful implementation as judged by different parties. In a relatively short time this will provide useful data for a more "research informed management" of these programmes.

A science is only as good as its research methods. The science of quality improvement is being developed by research into how changes to organisation and practice improve patient outcomes. However, insufficient attention has been given to methods for evaluating and understanding large scale programmes for improving quality. As these programmes are increasingly used, there is particular need for studies which not only assess their effectiveness, but also examine how best to implement them.

Key messages

- Much time and resources are expended on large scale quality improvement programmes such as a hospital quality programme, a national accreditation scheme, or a guidelines programme.
- We know little about how these programmes are actually implemented, how organization and behaviour are affected, about results, or about conditions for success.
- There are challenges in evaluating these complex changing interventions.
- There are evaluation methods which can be used to understand how these programmes are carried through, their results, and conditions for success.
- More research on these interventions could contribute to more effective quality programmes, less waste of time and money, and to developing the theoretical basis of quality improvement.

References

1 West E. Management matters: the link between hospital organisation and quality of patient care. *Qual Health Care* 2001;**10**:40–8.
2 Bigelow B, Arndt M. Total quality management: field of dreams. *Health Care Manage Rev* 1995;**20**:15–25.
3 Motwani J, Sower V, Brasier L. Implementing TQM in the health care sector. *Health Care Manage Rev* 1996;**21**:73–82.
4 Øvretveit J, Aslaksen A. *The quality journeys of six Norwegian hospitals*. Oslo: Norwegian Medical Association, 1999.
5 Shortell S, Bennet C, Byck G. Assessing the impact of continuous quality improvement on clinical practice: what will it take to accelerate progress. *Milbank Quarterly* 1998;**76**:593–624.
6 Blumenthal D, Kilo C. A report card on continuous quality improvement. *Milbank Quarterly* 1998;**76**:625–48.
7 Øvretveit J. The Norwegian approach to integrated quality development. *J Manage Med* 2001;**15**:125–41.
8 Shortell SM, O'Brien JL, Hughes EF, *et al*. Assessing the progress of TQM in US hospitals: findings from two studies. *Qual Lett Healthc Lead* 1994;**6**:14–17.
9 Shortell SM, O'Brien JL, Carman JM, *et al*. Assessing the impact of continuous quality improvement/total quality management: concept versus implementation *Health Serv Res* 1995;**30**:377–401.

10 Carman JM, Shortell SM, Foster, RW, *et al*. Keys for successful implementation of total quality management in hospitals. *Health Care Manage Rev* 1996;**21**:48–60.
11 Boerstler H, Foster RW, O'Connor EJ, *et al*. Implementation of total quality management: conventional wisdom versus reality. *Hospital Health Serv Admin* 1996;**41**:143–59.
12 Gustafson D, Hundt A. Findings of innovation research applied to quality management principles for health care. *Health Care Manage Rev* 1995;**20**:16–24.
13 Gustafson D, Risberg L, Gering D, *et al*. *Case studies from the quality improvement support system*. ACHPR Research Report 97-0022. Washington: US Department of Health and Human Services, 1997.
14 Shaw C. External assessment of health care. *BMJ* 2001;**322**:851–4.
15 Thompson R, McElroy H, Kazandjian V. Maryland hospital quality indicator project in the UK. *Qual Health Care* 1997;**6**:49–55.
16 Cleveland Health Quality Choice Program (CHQCP). Summary report from the Cleveland Health Quality Choice Program. *Qual Manage Health Care* 1995;**3**:78–90.
17 Rosenthal G, Harper D. Cleveland health quality choice. *Jt Comm J Qual Improv* 1994;**8**:425–42.
18 Pennsylvania Health Care Cost Containment Council (PHCCCC). *Hospital effectiveness report*. Harrisburg: Pennsylvania Health Care Cost Containment Council, 1992.
19 National Institute of Standards and Technology (NIST). *The Malcolm Baldridge national quality award 1990 application guidelines*. Gaithersburg, MD: National Institute of Standards and Technology, 1990.
20 Hertz H, Reimann C, Bostwick M. The Malcolm Baldridge National Quality Award concept: could it help stimulate or accelerate healthcare quality improvement? *Qual Manage Health Care* 1994;**2**:63–72.
21 European Foundation for Quality Management (EFQM). *The European Quality Award 1992*. Brussels: European Foundation for Quality Management, 1992.
22 Sweeney J, Heaton C. Interpretations and variations of ISO 9000 in acute health care. *Int J Qual Health Care* 2000;**12**:203–9.
23 Shaw C. External quality mechanisms for health care: summary of the ExPeRT project on visitatie, accreditation, EFQM and ISO assessment in European Union countries. *Int J Qual Health Care* 2000;**12**:169–75.
24 Øvretveit J. Quality assessment and comparative indicators in the Nordic countries. *Int J Health Planning Manage* 2001;**16**:229–41.
25 Wensing M, Grol R. Single and combined strategies for implementing changes in primary care: a literature review. *Int J Qual Health Care* 1994;**6**: 115–32.
26 Øvretveit J. How to run an effective improvement collaborative. *Int J Health Care Qual Assur* 2002;**15**:33–44.
27 Plsek P, Wilson T. Complexity science: complexity, leadership, and management in healthcare organisations. *BMJ* 2001;**323**:746–9.
28 Øvretveit J. Evaluating hospital quality programmes. *Evaluation* 1997;**3**:451–68.
29 Cook T, Campbell D. *Quasi-experimentation: design and analysis issues for field settings*. Chicago: Rand McNally, 1979.
30 Øvretveit J. *Action evaluation of health programmes and change: a handbook for a user focused approach*. Oxford: Radcliffe Medical Press, 2002.
31 Øvretveit J. *Evaluating health interventions*. Milton Keynes: Open University Press, 1998.
32 Yin R. *Case study research: design and methods*. Beverly Hills: Sage, 1994.

33 Jick T. Mixing qualitative and quantitative methods: triangulation in action. In: Van Maanen J, ed. *Qualitative methodology*. Beverly Hills: Sage, 1983.
34 Ferlie E, Gabbay J, FitzGerald F, *et al*. Evidence-based medicine and organisational change: an overview of some recent qualitative research. In: Mark A, Dopson S, eds. *Organisational behaviour in healthcare: the research agenda*. London: Macmillan, 1999.
35 Walshe K, Wallace L, Freeman T, *et al*. The external review of quality improvement in healthcare organisations: a qualitative study. *Int J Qual Health Care* 2001;**13**:367–74.
36 Øvretveit J. *Integrated quality development for public healthcare*. Oslo: Norwegian Medical Association, 1999.
37 Øvretveit J. The economics of quality: a practical approach. *Int J Health Care Qual Assur* 2000;**13**:200–7.
38 Rogers E. *Diffusion of innovation*. New York: Free Press, 1983.
39 Gustafson D, Cats-Baril W, Alemei F. *Systems to support health policy analysis*. Ann Arbor: Health Administration Press, University of Michigan, 1992.

9: Methods for evaluation of small scale quality improvement projects

GILL HARVEY, MICHEL WENSING

Evaluation is an integral component of quality improvement and there is much to be learned from the evaluation of small scale quality improvement initiatives at a local level. This type of evaluation is useful for a number of different reasons including monitoring the impact of local projects, identifying and dealing with issues as they arise within a project, comparing local projects to draw lessons, and collecting more detailed information as part of a bigger evaluation project. Focused audits and developmental studies can be used for evaluation within projects, while methods such as multiple case studies and process evaluations can be used to draw generalised lessons from local experiences and to provide examples of successful projects. Evaluations of small scale quality improvement projects help those involved in improvement initiatives to optimise their choice of interventions and use of resources. Important information to add to the knowledge base of quality improvement in health care can be derived by undertaking formal evaluation of local projects, particularly in relation to building theory around the processes of implementation and increasing understanding of the complex change processes involved.

Many questions can be raised about the impact of quality improvement programmes in health care. Do they work? How can they be improved? What factors promote or inhibit their success? What can we learn from our local experiences? Why do they work in some settings and not in others? Different research designs are needed depending on the focus of the specific question the research is trying to answer, often involving the setting up of an external research project. But what about quality improvement initiatives that take place on a small scale such as a local ward, unit, or departmental level: a clinical audit project, a process redesign effort or a unit that is participating in a breakthrough collaborative – should these be evaluated and, if so, how?

Evaluations of small scale quality improvement projects (defined as projects in a specific ward, unit, or practice) can help both those who undertake such projects and researchers of quality improvement interventions. An important first step in any evaluation is the clarification of its purpose. Evaluations of small scale projects may encompass one or more of the following aims:

1. to monitor the success or impact of a local quality improvement project over time – for example, to make sure the project is achieving the desired results and to demonstrate the impact of the project to others
2. to identify issues or problems as they arise within the project so that actions can be taken to change or redesign the project while it is in progress
3. to compare similarities and differences in a number of local projects to draw out common lessons learnt and develop hypotheses for future research
4. to collect more detailed information about the processes and outcomes of implementing a local quality improvement initiative as part of a bigger evaluation research project to help to explain the findings of this project.

Broadly speaking, the reasons for evaluation relate to two main types of learning – learning within the project (points 1 and 2 above) and more generalised learning about the implementation of quality improvement (points 3 and 4 above). The first type of learning is associated with the processes of clinical audit and quality improvement, while the second type is associated with research. This paper will outline a number of approaches and methods for the evaluation of quality improvement at a local level. Table 9.1 highlights the four main approaches that will be presented.

Table 9.1 Types of evaluations in small scale improvement projects

Research designs	Aims	Approaches
Focused audit studies	Monitor impact of the activities over time	Evaluation as a component of quality improvement
Developmental studies	Identify issues and intervene when necessary, develop hypotheses	Evaluation linked to action by participants in the case of action research
Multiple case studies	Draw lessons and develop hypotheses	Case reports and comparisons across a number of local projects
Process evaluations	Explain the findings of a bigger research project	In-depth analyses of projects as part of a bigger research project

Types of evaluations in small scale improvement projects

Focused audit studies

Local quality improvement projects typically involve implementing one or more specific changes that are designed to bring about improvements on a focused topic, such as a new way of treating a particular condition or a different way of organising delivery of care. Examples include a quality improvement project to ensure the provision of evidence-based pain management to patients following gastrointestinal surgery or a project to introduce more clinically and cost effective ways of organising patient centred stroke services at a district or regional level. Within projects such as these, evaluation should comprise an integral part of the quality improvement process linked to an explicit assessment of the effect of implementing planned changes in practice. For example, in models of continuous quality improvement the third phase of the plan–do–study–act cycle[1] involves collecting

Box 9.1 Role of evaluation within a project designed to improve the repeat prescribing process in a busy general practice setting[3]

This project was established within a general practice in the UK to improve the service to patients in relation to ordering repeat prescriptions. A 48 hour target for processing repeat prescriptions was set. A multiprofessional team was established to work on the quality improvement initiative, using continuous quality improvement methods and supported by an external facilitator. Following the steps of the plan–do–study–act cycle, the team began by gathering information to assess their current practice and plan the necessary changes. This included the preparation of flow charts of the repeat prescribing process, and a baseline audit over a one month period to assess how many prescriptions were actually ready for collection within 48 hours and to identify the number that required medical records to be checked before they could be signed.

Information gained from the flow charts and the initial audit results helped the team to identify those areas where they could introduce changes that would have the most impact and to identify the measures they would use to evaluate the change process. Once planned, the changes were implemented in practice and repeat audits were undertaken at 6, 12, and 24 months. The resulting data were presented in two main ways: a comparison of results at baseline, 6, 12, and 24 months; and graphs plotting the turnaround times for consecutive prescriptions over time.

Analysis of the results helped the team to understand more clearly what was happening. Although 95% of repeat prescriptions were available within 48 hours at the baseline audit, the graphs illustrated considerable variation which led to frustration among staff. Repeated audits demonstrated improvements in turnaround times, significant reductions in the number of records that needed to be checked, and much greater staff satisfaction as the process became more consistent and more effective.

data to evaluate whether changes introduced during the "do" phase have actually realised improvements in practice or patient care. Similarly, in models of clinical audit the process typically includes an audit cycle in which a key stage involves evaluating how practice compares with expected standards and implementing changes accordingly. These changes are then re-evaluated by a process of re-audit.[2] The example illustrated in Box 9.1 shows the role of evaluation within a project designed to improve the repeat prescribing process in a general practice setting.[3]

Measurements should be valid but simple.[4] Chart reviews, surveys among patients, or simple observations of events are all examples of possible data collection methods. The relative simplicity of the measurements is perhaps most visible in the absence of complex case mix adjustments, as these would often require extensive additional data collection. Audit studies may comprise sampling of cases, such as patient records, so that statistical techniques can be used to indicate the reliability of figures. Generalisation to a larger population of clinicians or practices is, however, not sought. Focused audit studies help to close the loop of the quality improvement cycle, an area where many projects have been shown to fail in the past.[5] Furthermore, information on the impact of the project aids learning from the local project, which is the aim of the approaches described next.

Developmental studies

Evaluation may also be beneficial with ongoing quality improvement projects to help assess what actions may be needed to refine or improve the design of the project, or specific interventions within the project. Evaluation mechanisms can be built into a local improvement project through both informal and formal methods. At an informal level, this might involve observation and discussion with colleagues about the process of how the project is going. Alternatively, the evaluation may employ a more formal developmental research method, particularly where there is a need to provide support, feedback, or help to the project team.[6] One method is action research, which is broadly defined as an approach to research that actively involves participants and which has an explicit focus on promoting and facilitating change.[7] It is an approach that has been used in a range of healthcare settings in the UK and has been the subject of a recent review to define the approach more clearly and assess its impact in practice.[8] From this review a number of factors key to the success of action research were highlighted, including participation, maintaining a "real world" focus, resources, and project management.

Developmental approaches to evaluation may be particularly useful within the context of organisational learning[9] and learning by professionals[10] because of their action orientated approach and the focus on personal and

Box 9.2 An action research approach to introduce new wound management practices in a community nursing organisation[11]

This project was set up to establish and encourage an improved approach to wound management in a community nursing organisation in South Australia. Within the organisation about 50% of client visits were related to wound care, hence the importance of promoting best practice in this area of care. Following an initial survey of wound management practices, participatory action research groups were established to address some of the issues identified.

Each group followed an action research approach with its three phases of planning, action, and evaluation being undertaken as part of a cyclical process. Volunteers were sought for the participatory action research groups, and core principles of action research including the group's responsibility for agenda setting, decision making about appropriate actions, and reaching consensus were emphasised. One group elected to focus specifically on evidence-based practice relating to the care of leg ulcers, particularly appropriate methods for cleansing chronic leg ulcers. This involved comparing the use of tap water cleansing to an aseptic technique with sterile saline solution.

As part of the planning phase, an initial review of the literature was undertaken which highlighted the fact that the evidence base underpinning cleansing practice was limited and inconclusive. However, from this review and their own clinical experience, the group reached the conclusion that there was no evidence to suggest that tap water cleansing was ineffective. It also had the advantage of being more cost effective. Moving on to the action phase of the research cycle, the group examined the current cleansing practices used by their colleagues and reasons underpinning their chosen approach. This highlighted concerns around infection influencing the choice of the aseptic technique, so the group ran educational sessions to disseminate the research evidence on cleansing wounds. A repeat survey was subsequently carried out which showed an increase in the use of the clean tap water technique. As a spin-off from the action research and the identification of a lack of evidence to inform cleansing practices, a randomised controlled trial was subsequently set up to compare the use of warmed sterile saline with warm tap water for cleansing chronic leg ulcers.

professional development. Within a quality improvement project, developmental research may form part of a flexible intervention programme – for example, a tailored educational approach to implement clinical guidelines, enabling actions to be planned on the basis of insight into the barriers for change. Box 9.2 illustrates the use of action research to introduce new wound management practices in a community nursing organisation.[11] This example also illustrates the use of a focused audit to assess the impact of the project as an integral part of the study design. The type of knowledge generated by developmental approaches is seen to be practical and propositional,[8] and the focus is on generating and refining interpretations through inductive processes within repeated cycles of action research. As quality improvement projects studied through action research do not usually involve random or purposeful sampling, the generalisability of the knowledge generated may be limited to associations between different variables within the project under study.

Multiple case studies

In the approaches described above the focus has mainly been on learning within and about individual quality improvement projects. However, to draw out common experiences and lessons for the purpose of more generalised learning about quality improvement, it is most helpful to compare experiences across a number of local improvement projects to identify similarities and differences. This presents particular challenges in terms of identifying an appropriate research methodology for a number of reasons.

- Each local project may be focused on a different topic for improvement and have different targets.
- There may be considerable variation in the processes of implementation as well as external influences across sites – for example, reasons for introducing the quality improvement initiative, membership of the quality improvement team, use of an internal/external facilitator or change agent.
- Process and outcome indicators used to audit the progress and impact of the project are likely to be specific to each individual site.

Dealing with these context specific issues requires an approach that is able to take account of local differences yet can still compare across projects to draw out some more generalisable findings. One approach often used in these situations is the multiple case or comparative case study method.[12,13]

Box 9.3 Key steps in the comparative case study approach

- Select individual cases relevant to the issues to be studied.
- Collect data within individual sites using a range of quantitative and qualitative methods.
- Analyse the data within individual sites using appropriate quantitative and qualitative methods of analysis – for example, descriptive statistics, thematic analysis of qualitative data.
- Compare data analyses across sites to draw more general conclusions and/or generate hypotheses for further testing.

Increasingly, the comparative case study approach is being applied in health care, notably within the field of evidence-based practice and quality improvement. Here the focus is often on "why" questions, such as "why and under what conditions clinical professionals decide to adopt an innovation or change their clinical practice".[13] Recently published studies addressing questions such as this include an evaluation of the impact of guidelines on the management of adult asthma,[14] the uptake of evidence-based practice in elective orthopaedics,[15] the management of glue ear,[16] an evaluation of the "Promoting Action on Clinical Effectiveness" initiative across 16 sites in England,[17] and an evaluation of the six projects forming the Welsh Clinical Effectiveness National Demonstration Project.[18] Box 9.3 summarises some of the key steps involved in the comparative case study approach.

Purposeful selection of cases to be included in the study contributes to its validity because a relevant diversity of cases is studied.[13,15] In reality, however, the range of cases studied may be determined by what cases are available. The case study approach is not characterised by one specific method for data collection. Instead, a key feature is the use of data from a range of sources which are often collected using both quantitative and qualitative methods – for example, questionnaire surveys, semi-structured interviews, written documents, and direct observations. Combining data from multiple sources to study specific variables (known as "triangulation") is recommended as it increases the validity of the data.[19] It may, however, be expensive or impossible to achieve triangulation for all the variables studied.

The data analysis in multiple case studies is not characterised by one specific technique but by its overall approach. It is recognised that the cases are heterogeneous, so the analysis usually takes two approaches. Firstly, the cases are described in depth – comparable to detailed case reports of complex patients – including, for instance, both factual descriptions and the views of the participants. A systematic approach may then be used to derive lessons from such case reports – for instance, by verifying ideas on cases other than the one on which the idea was originally based.[20] Secondly, multiple case studies can be used to examine associations between variables and hypotheses on determinants of success, although formal statistical testing may be impossible. This requires that information on the impact of the projects is available from, for instance, focused audit studies.

Box 9.4 describes a project in which a number of hypotheses were developed a priori and then tested on the basis of the data available. Testing hypotheses is only valid for a limited number of predefined factors; if too many factors are studied, some associations will be found by chance. The associations found should be interpreted as hypothesis generating rather than testing. Although the heterogeneity of cases means that data cannot be pooled by more traditional methods such as systematic reviews or meta-analyses, case study researchers are testing methodological approaches to pool results across similar studies. For example, Dopson and colleagues[22] reported an attempt to pool data across a suite of seven related studies examining the diffusion of innovations in health care. This involved a multi-staged approach to critically review and summarise the findings of individual studies before identifying themes that were common across the studies. These themes were then verified by independent analysis of the data, followed by collective discussion and simultaneous analysis.

Process evaluations

Methods used for the in-depth study of local projects can also be helpful when undertaking evaluations of quality improvement initiatives using other research designs which explicitly aim at generalised knowledge. For example, a randomised controlled trial (RCT) may be set up to evaluate

Box 9.4 Multiple case study approach to evaluate the implementation of 10 programmes to increase physical exercise in older adults[21]

Physical exercise improves the health status of adults, including older adults, but many adults perform very little physical exercise. A range of programmes in the Netherlands which focus on walking, dancing, and aerobics aim to encourage older adults to become physically active for at least 30 minutes per day, at least five days a week. The clinical effectiveness of many of these programmes has been proven, so the focus is now on effective implementation in terms of setting up programmes and optimal participation of older adults in these programmes.

A multiple case study project has been undertaken to evaluate the implementation of 10 physical exercise programmes. This study has taken two approaches. Firstly, structured descriptions of the programmes were made and showed, for instance, that a variety of methods were used to improve participation in the programmes such as personal contact in case of absence, obligatory indication of check-out, and provision of drinks to enhance social interaction. Furthermore, project leaders were asked to describe the most important barriers and facilitators to the success of the programme. Many mentioned, for example, the problem of convincing municipalities and welfare organisations of the relevance of the programme. These data were used to make structured descriptions of the cases.

Secondly, the study team proposed about 25 hypotheses on factors that influenced the success of implementation. For instance, it was hypothesised that the programme was more successful if there was a local tradition of collaboration between different organisations and if the physical exercise was three times a week (rather than five). Structured questionnaires were distributed to individuals involved in organising or delivering the programmes to collect data on the variables indicated by the hypotheses. Where possible, information on the success of implementation was derived from evaluations within the projects. These data were used to test the predefined hypotheses. The results indicated that successful implementation of physical exercise programmes was associated with larger investment by organisations in the programme, a prevailing view that audit and evaluation were relevant, and a local tradition of innovation in health-care services. Although the number of cases is usually much lower than the number of variables, defining hypotheses a priori provides some protection against associations found by chance.

the effectiveness of a particular approach to quality improvement. Within the design of the RCT, the research team may decide to collect more detailed qualitative data from a sample of the study sites involved in the trial to examine more fully what happens during the implementation process. This, in turn, may inform their subsequent understanding of the relationships between process and outcome data and provide information that helps to explain the trial findings in more detail. Another aim may be to provide examples of successful sites ("success stories") that can be used to disseminate the message of the trial to a wider audience. A potential problem that needs to be considered, however, is the effect that additional measurements (collected as part of the in-depth evaluation) may have on the subjects participating in the quality improvement project, as these may be undesirable in the context of a controlled trial. If this is the case, it is important to find the right balance between learning about the programme and avoiding the test effect. Process evaluations of quality improvement have been discussed in detail in Chapter 11.

Discussion

All practitioners of quality improvement need to know the impact of specific programmes and possible ways to improve their effectiveness. Focused audit studies and developmental studies are designs that can help to structure these evaluations and provide information to determine the optimal choice of interventions and use of resources for quality improvement. Although the generalisability of the findings may be limited to the programmes evaluated, such evaluations can help to shed light on the more promising quality improvement methods and approaches.

An issue which is often debated is the extent to which clinicians and others who undertake quality improvement projects at a local level should use rigorous evaluation methods. For instance, how many cases should they study to get a reliable figure, should they adjust for case mix severity, and how extensive should the data collection on each case be? From a research point of view it is tempting to promote the use of rigorous approaches, but we believe that it is not realistic or necessary to evaluate each and every quality improvement project with the same level of rigour required by research. Simple evaluations can help to identify the methods that are most acceptable to clinical staff and appear to result in change of clinical performance. The probability that effective methods will be rejected on the basis of such evaluations appears to be small because rigorous evaluations such as randomised trials usually show smaller (and not larger) effects than simple evaluations.

Evaluations of small scale projects can also contribute to more generalised learning and inform scientific knowledge about quality improvement in health care. They can help to provide insight into causality if some sort of control is included in the design. A randomised trial is the ideal type of evaluation, but it is inefficient to trial interventions before they have been proved to be promising in small scale evaluation (Chapter 7). This is particularly relevant for organisational and structural changes which require large scale expensive trials. Multiple case studies may be particularly useful for testing the relevance of factors associated with a programme or its organisational context. Process evaluations help to understand the mechanism of causality better and contribute to the evidence on a specific intervention in this way. From a research perspective, these two designs can be used for studies that are equivalent to early phase studies in pharmaceutical research and are performed before large clinical trials.[23]

Conclusions

Implementing change is complex and the processes involved are still not fully understood. Quality improvement projects are undertaken in many different settings and the knowledge gained from these projects is important to help increase our understanding of implementing effective change. It is useful to distinguish between evaluation undertaken to enable learning within the project and evaluation that aims to contribute to more generalised learning and inform scientific knowledge about quality improvement in health care. The appropriate methodology for evaluation needs to be elaborated, as not all interventions can or need to be tested in controlled trials.[24] A range of methods can be applied to evaluate small scale improvement projects, including focused audit studies, developmental research, multiple case studies, and process evaluations within RCTs. These approaches are characterised by their overall research approach rather than by the specific techniques for data collection or data analysis. Further development of the methodology for evaluation of small scale improvement projects is recommended.

Key messages

- Focused audits of the impact of local quality improvement projects help those involved to learn from the project.
- In-depth study of local projects using developmental approaches to evaluation, case study methodology, or process evaluations can provide important insight into how and why programmes work in practice.
- These evaluations are characterised by their overall approach rather than by the use of specific techniques for sampling, data collection, or data analysis.
- Further development of the methodology for evaluation of local quality improvement projects is recommended.

References

1 Langley GJ, Nolan KM, Norman CL, Provost LP, Nolan TW. *The improvement guide*. San Francisco: Jossey-Bass, 1996.
2 Morrell C, Harvey G. *The clinical audit handbook: improving the quality of health care*. London: Ballière Tindall, 1999.
3 Cox S, Wilcock P, Young J. Improving the repeat prescribing process in a busy general practice. A study using continuous quality improvement methodology. *Qual Health Care* 1999;**8**:119–25.
4 Solberg LI, Mosser G, McDonald S. The three faces of performance measurement: improvement, accountability and research. *Jt Comm J Qual Improv* 1997;**23**:135–47.
5 Johnston G, Crombie IK, Davies HTO, *et al*. Reviewing audit: barriers and facilitating factors for effective clinical audit. *Qual Health Care* 2000;**9**:23–36.
6 Øvretveit J. *Evaluating health interventions*. Buckingham: Open University Press, 1998.
7 Lewin K. Frontiers in group dynamics: social planning and action research. *Human Relations* 1947;**1**:143–53.
8 Waterman H, Tillen D, Dickson R, *et al*. Action research: a systematic review and guidance for assessment. *Health Technol Assess* 2001;**5**(23).
9 Argyris C. *On organisational learning*. Cambridge, MA: Blackwell Business, 1992.
10 Schon DA. *Educating the reflective practitioner*. London: Jossey-Bass, 1988.
11 Selim P, Bashford C, Grossman C. Evidence-based practice: tap water cleansing of leg ulcers in the community. *J Clin Nurs* 2001;**10**:372–9.
12 Yin RK. *Case study research: design and methodology*. London: Sage, 1989.
13 Fitzgerald L. Case studies as a research tool. *Qual Health Care* 1999;**8**:75.
14 Dawson S, Sutherland K, Dopson S, *et al*. Changing clinical practice: views about the management of adult asthma. *Qual Health Care* 1999;**8**:253–61.

15 Ferlie E, Wood M, Fitzgerald L. Some limits to evidence-based medicine: a case study from elective orthopaedics. *Qual Health Care* 1999;**8**:99–107.
16 Dopson S, Miller R, Dawson S, *et al.* Influences on clinical practice: the case of glue ear. *Qual Health Care* 1999;**8**:108–18.
17 Dopson S, Gabbay J, Locock L, *et al.* Evaluation of the PACE programme. In: Understanding the role of opinion leaders in improving clinical effectiveness. *Soc Sci Med* 2001;**53**:745–57.
18 Locock L, Chambers D, Surender R, *et al.* Evaluation of the Welsh clinical effectiveness initiative national demonstration project. In: Understanding the role of opinion leaders in improving clinical effectiveness. *Soc Sci Med* 2001;**53**:745–57.
19 Shih FJ. Triangulation in nursing research: issues of conceptual clarity and purpose. *J Adv Nurs* 1998;**28**:631–41.
20 Miles MB, Huberman AM. *Qualitative data analysis. A sourcebook of new methods.* London: Sage, 1984.
21 Laurant M, Harmsen M, Wensing M. *Effective implementation of physical exercise programmes for older adults.* Nijmegen: Centre for Quality of Care Research, 2001.
22 Dopson S, Fitzgerald L, Ferlie E, *et al.* No magic targets! Changing clinical practice to become more evidence based. *Health Care Manage Rev* 2002;**27**:35–47.
23 Freemantle N, Wood J, Crawford F. Evidence into practice, experimentation and quasi experimentation: are the methods up to the task? *J Epidemiol Community Health* 1998;**52**:75–81.
24 Black N. Why do we need observational studies to evaluate the effectiveness of health care. *BMJ* 1996;**312**:1215–8.

10: Designing a quality improvement intervention: a systematic approach

MARLOES VAN BOKHOVEN, GERJO KOK, TRUDY VAN DER WEIJDEN

Most quality improvement or change management interventions are currently designed intuitively and their results are often disappointing. While improving the effectiveness of interventions requires systematic development, no specific methodology for composing intervention strategies and programmes is available. This chapter describes the methodology of systematically designing quality of care improvement interventions, including problem analysis, intervention design and pretests. Several theories on quality improvement and change management are integrated and valuable materials from health promotion are added. One method of health promotion – intervention mapping – is introduced and applied. It describes the translation of knowledge about barriers to and facilitators of change into a concrete intervention programme. Systematic development of interventions, although time consuming, appears to be worthwhile. Decisions that have to be made during the design process of a quality improvement intervention are visualised, allowing them to serve as a starting point for a systematic evaluation of the intervention.

Many different interventions have been developed to enhance the implementation of research findings or innovations in daily practice and to change professional or team performance. The Cochrane Effective Practice and Organisation of Care (EPOC) group have summarized their effects in several reviews and conclude that the effectiveness of most interventions is heterogeneous and limited, although combined and multifaceted efforts are generally more promising.[1,2] Explanations for these disappointing results include the difficulty of changing existing practice, non-optimal choices of intervention strategies, and the use of inadequate methods to design and evaluate interventions.[3–5] The use of rigorous research methods in quality improvement has now been generally accepted for evaluation of interventions, and increasingly also for the problem analysis of the healthcare topic that is to be changed. However, a scientific approach should also be accepted for the design process of the intervention. In the current situation, many developers of interventions tend to select their strategies intuitively, usually based on their familiarity with a specific strategy. The choice of the format of an intervention often precedes the choice of its contents. However, it is generally accepted that, to be effective, interventions should be targeted at specific barriers to and facilitators of change.[4,6,7] Systematic development of interventions and tailoring their content and format to the specific features of a target group and setting seems necessary to improve the effectiveness of patient care.

Steps to improve quality of care have been described as a cyclical process (Figure 10.1).[6,8,9] While the problem analysis step has been specified in the literature by several authors,[6,10,11] the literature on quality improvement research so far provides little information on the systematic translation of knowledge about barriers to and facilitators of change into concrete quality improvement interventions. This chapter focuses on the methodology of designing and pretesting such interventions. It addresses the question of how to link an intervention to the target problem in a transparent way. Several theories are described, both from the field of quality improvement and change management and from that of health promotion. As an example we use a quality improvement project on the problem of unnecessary laboratory test ordering by GPs in cases of medical uncertainty for which we have developed an intervention.

Problem analysis

Ideally, problem analysis precedes the design of an intervention. This analysis begins by describing the healthcare problem to be addressed in quantifiable measures, followed by the barriers to and facilitators of change, and then the target population.

Problem/target for improvement

Problem analysis

- Describe problems in quantifiable measures of quality of life, health, and quality of care
- Describe barriers and facilitators, both personal and in the external context
- Describe target population in terms of subgroups, stages of change

Design of intervention

- Specify intervention objectives
  - State expected changes in behaviour and external context
  - Specify performance objectives
  - Specify barrier s and facilitators
  - Create matrices of intervention objectives
- Select methods and strategies
  - Brainstorm on methods
  - Translate methods into practical strategies
  - Organise methods and strategies at each level
- Design the programme
  - Operationalise strategies into plans, considering implementers and sites
  - Develop and design documents
  - Produce programme materials

Pretest

- Testing materials
- Pilot test
- (Randomised) trial

- readability and usefulness of materials
- acceptability for target population
- understanding of messages
- coherence of programme
- feasibility of time schedule
- effectiveness of programme

Adoption and implementation

- Write implementation plan
- Implementation

Evaluation

- Write evaluation plan with effect measures and process measures
- Evaluate

Adjustment

Figure 10.1 Design process for quality of care improvement interventions

Describing the problem

Careful targeting of the intervention requires that the situation that is to be improved by the intervention is very clear. Several methods are available for the collection of data on processes, outcomes, and costs. It is advisable to take small but representative samples of professionals, patients, or written data, to use both quantitative and qualitative designs, and to fit the measurements into daily routines as much as possible.[12] The ultimate goal of every intervention is to improve the health and quality of life of patients or to maintain high standards of quality at lower costs. The intended improvement of health, quality of life, and quality of care should therefore be described in quantifiable terms, and standards of good quality of care should have been set.[13,14]

Identifying barriers to and facilitators of change

In tailoring the intervention, the next step is to identify barriers to and facilitators of change. Figure 10.2 presents a modified combined model based on the PRECEDE–PROCEED concept and the theory of planned behaviour,[15,16] showing different types of potential barriers and facilitators and the way in which they can influence professional behaviour and quality of life. Barriers and facilitators may be located within the person of the professional or in his or her external context.[7] Factors inherent in the professional – such as attitudes, perceived social influence, and self-efficacy – stimulate the intention to change, while skills are needed for actual change. Context factors can have different levels. External influence can come from other individuals (interpersonal level) – for example, a patient requesting treatment – but also from a larger group such as a nursing team (organisational level), a local professional society (community level), or a whole nation (societal level) – for example, through legislation or insurances. Major factors at the organisational level include the organisation's mission, goals, policies, procedures, structures, technologies, physical setting, collaboration, and resources.[17,18] At the community level, barriers and facilitators include collective self-efficacy, political efficacy, and motivation to act.[19] At the societal level changes take place through political influence. Factors

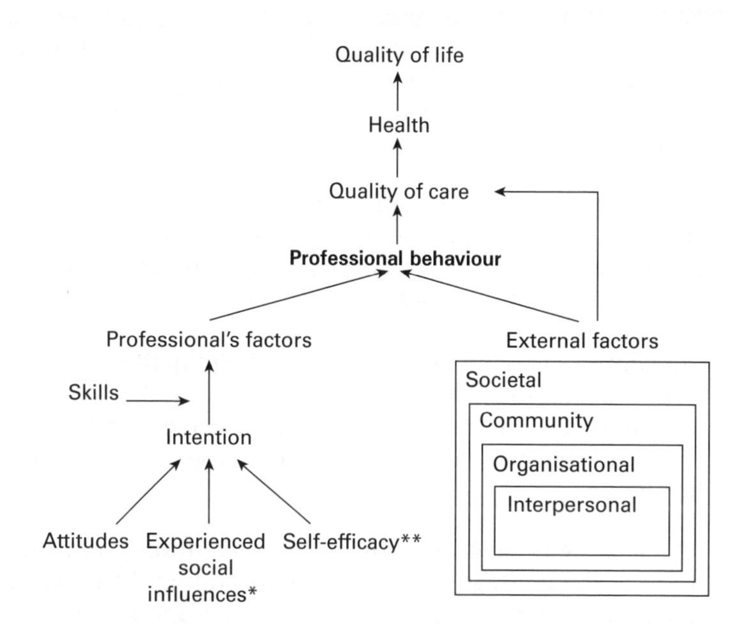

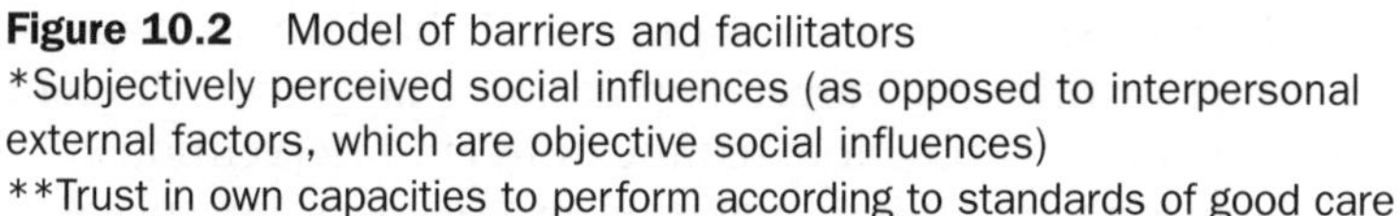

Figure 10.2 Model of barriers and facilitators
*Subjectively perceived social influences (as opposed to interpersonal external factors, which are objective social influences)
**Trust in own capacities to perform according to standards of good care

influencing the political decision process include the place where policies are made – whether outside or within the government, or within the government but requiring support from outside for passage[20] – and groups influencing the policy makers such as professional societies or patient groups.[21] The barriers and facilitators at different levels can be identified by detailed qualitative analysis of a few situations followed by quantitative studies among professionals, patients, and institutions to find out the relative importance of the various factors. Such studies can use questionnaires, interviews, and observations.[22]

Describing the target population

A third component of problem analysis is the description of the target population in terms of aspects influencing the change process such as the information channels they use. One aspect of the target population that needs to be clarified is the "stage of behavioural change". Behavioural changes in individuals (both at the personal and the interpersonal level) usually take place in a particular order.[10,11,23,24] Prochaska identified five stages.

1. Pre-contemplation: the target population is not aware that their behaviours should and can be improved.
2. Contemplation: the target population reflects on the advantages and disadvantages of changing their behaviours.
3. Preparation: concrete plans for change are made.
4. Action: changing behaviour starts.
5. Maintenance: the target population decides whether to continue the new behaviour or to relapse to the former behaviour.

Each stage sets specific goals for interventions: drawing attention to the message in stage 1, understanding the message in stage 2, changing barriers and facilitators in stage 3, changing behaviour in stage 4, and maintaining behaviour in stage 5. Subgroups within the target population may have different characteristics and therefore require different interventions.

Change at the organisational level also seems to take place in a particular order. Goodman et al[17] have identified seven stages.

1. Noticing the problem.
2. Searching for possible responses.
3. Evaluating alternatives.
4. Deciding to adopt a course of action based on a selected number of responses.
5. Initiating action within the system, which requires policy changes and resources necessary for implementation.
6. Implementation, including some organisation members changing their work behaviours and relationships.
7. Institutionalising the change, which means including it in strategic plans, job descriptions, and budgets so that it becomes a routine part of organisational operations.

Such distinctions between stages of change may be very important as the key actors at which the intervention is targeted can vary depending of the stage of change.[25] Thus, in the earlier stages senior level staff are the target population

Box 10.1 Example of problem analysis[26–29]

General practitioners frequently see patients with unexplained complaints. The complaints are usually self-limiting and the value of blood testing is nil due to the low pretest probability of disease. For this reason, a national guideline recommends postponing blood testing in this category of patients by one month. Nevertheless, many GPs request several blood tests immediately, which might have negative effects such as unnecessary further investigations, fear in patients, somatization, and high costs. The goal of the intervention is to stimulate GPs to adhere to the national guideline.

A qualitative study was performed to collect information on the barriers and facilitators influencing the test requesting behaviour. Consultations by the GPs were observed and field notes were taken on a pre-structured form. Afterwards, GPs were interviewed about barriers to and facilitators of test ordering behaviour for "unexplained complaints" in a non-pre-structured way. This was followed by a search of the literature on possible barriers and facilitators. A questionnaire survey of GPs was then carried out which more specifically dealt with different types of barriers and facilitators, with questions on experiences with changing behaviour, opinions about the value of blood testing, perceived social influence from patients and colleagues or others on test ordering, grading their own capacities to change test ordering behaviour, and interest in postgraduate education. GPs were also asked to rate their stage of change regarding consultation skills and test requesting behaviour.

Since many GPs reported experiencing pressure from patients to do laboratory tests, a short questionnaire survey was held among patients in the waiting room before they consulted their GPs. Patients were asked questions about what they thought their GPs could do for them. No further research was done at the other external levels because successful interventions on test requesting behaviour at those levels had already been implemented before, so there was not much room for improvement. In addition, as many GPs work in single person practices, the external level (organisational and societal) in Dutch general practice has less impact than, for example, in hospitals.

Some examples of the barriers and facilitators found are presented below:

- Attitudes
  - Blood testing does not have harmful effects
  - Blood testing is a more efficient strategy than explaining a wait and see policy
- Perceived social influences
  - Patients expect blood testing
  - Patients are anxious

(Continued)

Box 10.1 *(Continued)*

- Self-efficacy
  - Perceived capability to resist pressure from patients
  - Difficulty of postponing testing when under pressure of time
- Skills
  - Routines (non-conscious skills)
  - Communication skills
  - Diagnostic skills (doing laboratory tests instead of physical examination)
- External factors
  - Exaggerated expectations of tests among patients
  - Lack of knowledge about limitations of tests among patients

where decisions are made to start the change process, and also at the final stage where the decision is made whether to institutionalise the change or not. Mid-level staff are important during the adoption and early implementation stages, in which skills to introduce procedures and provide training on the innovation are critical. In the adoption stage, the people who have to apply the change in their daily professional practice form the target population of the intervention.

An example of problem analysis is given in Box 10.1.

The actual design process

Based on the findings of the problem analysis, the actual design process can start. The steps described below have been derived from the "intervention mapping" theory, a method for designing interventions originally aimed at unhealthy behaviours[30,31] that appeared to be helpful.

Specification of performance and intervention objectives

This step focuses on linking barriers and facilitators found in the problem analysis to concrete behaviours of professionals and on deriving objectives for quality improvement from this relation. It is always people who play a crucial role in managing change, even at the external level. This step therefore begins with reframing both problem behaviours and external causes found in the problem analysis into desirable behaviours in practice – performance objectives such as "GP discusses a one month 'wait and see' policy in consultations with patients presenting unexplained complaints" or "national college of GPs disseminates guideline to all GPs". These performance objectives need to be specific and measurable in order to tailor the intervention to the heart of the problem and to be able to evaluate the effects of the intervention later. In addition, the frequency of the behaviours and the situations in which they should be performed are specifically described (Table 10.1, column 1). Goals may include not only changing behaviour but also maintaining behaviour.[32] As a check it might be important to ask members of the target population and service providers by interviews or questionnaires, for example, whether they consider the objective important for achieving the improvement.

Achieving the performance objectives requires the barriers and facilitators to be influenced. Many barriers and facilitators are usually found and, since it is impossible to target an intervention to all of these, a selection has to be made. Two criteria for selecting barriers and facilitators are "importance" and "changeability". If a barrier or facilitator is not important, efforts to change it do not make sense – for example, a "wait and see" policy of one month is cheaper than immediate blood testing in patients with unexplained complaints as most complaints are self limiting within one month. However, GPs consider costs to be only a minor factor in determining their behaviour so it is not useful to design an intervention providing information about costs to GPs. The same applies to changeability – for example, GPs consider a lack of time per consultation as an important reason for requesting blood tests instead of explaining to patients the limited use of testing which is more time consuming. The time scheduled per consultation, however, can hardly be changed as it is based on national rules. Sometimes information about importance and changeability can be extracted from the literature or from the quantitative research executed in the problem analysis phase.

Performance objectives (Table 10.1, column 1) and selected barriers and facilitators (Table 10.1, row 1) can next be linked in a matrix, allowing a concrete intervention objective to be

Table 10.1 Example of part of a matrix with intervention objectives for GPs

	Barriers and facilitators		
Performance objectives	**High outcome expectation of tests**	**Lack of communication skills**	**Uncertainty of GP**
Performs adequate history taking and physical examination	GP states that physical examination is a way of taking patients' complaints seriously	GP asks patients about reasons for encounter and chooses formulation which he/she feels most comfortable with	GP states that testing does not yield more information than performing physical examination
Explains findings and conclusions to patient appropriately	GP states the importance of explaining findings and conclusions to patient	GP demonstrates the use of different formulations to explain findings from history taking and physical examination to patients	GP shows patients he/she is convinced that findings from history taking and examination are sufficient to feel reassured
Discusses a one month "wait and see" policy	–	GP uses instruction materials in addition to verbal message	GP shows awareness that his/her own uncertainty is a reason to request blood tests

In the matrix three performance objectives for GPs (left column) are set against a selection of three barriers and facilitators (top row). The cells show the resulting intervention objectives. If the achievement of a performance objective does not require a barrier or facilitator to be addressed by the intervention, the cell at their intersection remains empty.

formulated in each cell of the matrix (Table 10.1, cells). For example, in order to achieve the goal of having GPs use adequate history taking and physical examination in practice (performance objective), the intervention should address barriers such as "uncertainty of GP" so that, as a result of the intervention, the GP "states that laboratory testing does not yield more information than physical examination" (intervention objective). In the example shown in Table 10.1 only some of the barriers have been worked out. In addition, the problem analysis revealed that patients have high pre-consultation expectations of laboratory tests and demand tests, which influences the behaviour of GPs. The intervention was therefore also targeted at the patients. As patients require a different intervention from GPs, their goals and their barriers and facilitators were entered into a different matrix which is not shown here. As stated above, we decided not to target the intervention at other external levels.

Like performance objectives, intervention objectives are formulated in terms of measurable behaviours, but intervention objectives are the aims of the intervention programme rather than the aims of performance in daily practice. If the problem analysis reveals that there are target populations at more than one level or that different subgroups in the target population require different interventions, separate matrices should be drawn up for every group. Interventions may thus be targeted at different people or organisations including assistants, patients, practice teams, hospital departments, politicians, and insurance companies.

Selection of methods and strategies

Once concrete intervention objectives have been defined, one can start searching for concrete methods and strategies for achieving these objectives. A good start is to have a brainstorming session in an expert group and to make a provisional list of potential methods and strategies. Who is "expert" depends on the problem for which an intervention is being developed and may include members of the target population. The list can be extended by a literature search using resources such as the EPOC database.[33] To enable a broad search, three approaches to searching literature databases are recommended.

1. By medical or health care subject – for example, "laboratory testing" or "unexplained complaints". The Cochrane Library includes several useful systematic reviews of interventions aimed at various topics.[33] Descriptive studies delineating variants of a service can also be of value.[3]
2. By concepts from the provisional list of methods and strategies or the barriers, facilitators, and behavioural objectives from the previous step – for example, "explanation of findings to patients" or "uncertainty".
3. By known theories – for example, goal setting theory or community organisation theory, or taxonomy of known strategies as used by the EPOC group. It is advisable to use this search strategy after the other strategies have been used to enable a broad focus on a number of methods.

If it is not only the personal or interpersonal levels that are important, databases from business or political sciences can be used to extend the search. Overviews of methods can be found in several books and papers on health promotion, quality improvement, and implementation of guidelines.[31,34] Objectives, methods, and strategies found can then be listed and the conditions under which they are effective can be added. Once sufficient methods have been collected, a selection can be made (Box 10.2).

Programme design

The result of the previous step is a list of methods and strategies which can be integrated into a coherent intervention. This requires a creative process. Brainstorming about possible intervention components and materials may be a good start. Interesting materials may have come up during the search of the literature for methods and strategies. However, in translating the methods and strategies into intervention components, several conditions should be kept in mind. For example, different "segments" of the target population may require different strategies, and the stages of behavioural change in the target population, and communication variables, are important for the order and format of the components of the intervention.[24] Different stages of the change process may require different messages

Box 10.2 Example of theories and strategies illustrating the search for theories on test ordering skills and the related barriers and facilitators

(1) Brainstorming session

- Strategies about skills training such as stepwise explanation of complex skills, giving opportunities to practise both in a laboratory situation and in practice.

(2) Literature search

- Search on "unexplained complaints" and related topics such as "irritable bowel syndrome", yielding papers on methods of cognitive behavioural therapy.
- Search on concepts such as "communication skills", adding methods such as "providing knowledge about skills", "attention to both skills and self-efficacy", and "offering coping strategies for difficult situations".
- Search on general theories applicable to skills changes: "rewarding systems", "goal setting theory", and "giving feedback".

(3) Pragmatic selection of methods and strategies

- Limiting conditions included the fact that group activities should take place in a safe environment where one is allowed to make mistakes.

and different modes of transmission. According to McGuire,[24] interventions should have a striking "appearance" to attract attention, while actually getting people to change depends more on the cogency of the message.

Another important condition is the opportunity to implement the intervention in daily practice as mentioned by Grol et al[7] Limiting factors in this respect include budget, human resources, available time, existing intervention formats, and characteristics of the organization that actually implements the intervention.

Pretest

Before the intervention can be implemented it is recommended to do a pretest. Pretests can consist of several stages, each of which can reveal information that requires adjustment of the intervention programme. The first stage involves testing the separate materials such as leaflets or course books. Such testing can be done by means of "technical" methods like readability formulae and tests of understanding, or by asking experts and members of the target population to try out the materials and to give their opinions, preferably using qualitative methods. A combination of approaches is advisable. The second stage involves running the intervention programme in a pilot group to test its coherence and the time schedule and to get an impression of its acceptability in the target population. Again, the evaluation of this stage should be done mainly by qualitative methods. The final stage before large scale implementation involves testing the intervention for its effectiveness on a smaller scale. The best method to evaluate its effectiveness is usually a randomised clinical trial. Variables can be extracted from the problem analysis while process measures such as those concerning participation rates should also be collected at this stage.

A possible intervention programme targeted at different levels is shown in Box 10.3.

Discussion

It is generally accepted that systematic development of quality improvement interventions is needed if such interventions are to be effective. Interventions should have the correct objectives, be targeted at the barriers and facilitators related to achieving the desired performance, and have programme components and materials adapted to specific objectives, target populations, barriers, and facilitators. In addition, it may be necessary to target the intervention not only at individual professionals but also at external factors which influence professional behaviour and the quality of care. The approach is ideally theory driven.

Several authors have described phases of the intervention design process: Green and Kreuter have described a problem analysis (PRECEDE) and evaluation (PROCEED) of interventions,[15] and McGuire has described the requirements of educational messages and materials given the stage of the change process.[24] However, no integrated approach to the design process from the perspective of the intervention

Box 10.3 Possible intervention programme targeted at different levels

The intervention goals are shown in brackets. The intervention was limited to the level of GPs and patients.

GPs
- Educational group meetings providing information, learning from peers, skills training and feedback (repetition of messages, improvement of information uptake, knowledge enhancement, problem awareness, attitude change, self-efficacy enhancement, skills improvement)
- Practice visit by expert (repetition of messages, tailoring of messages to individual's stage of change)
- Goal setting for try-out in GP's own practice (to stimulate actual practising)
- Introduction of materials to offer to patients (to reduce "empty hands feeling" among GPs, self-efficacy enhancement)

Patients
- Video message in waiting room (awareness of problem, knowledge enhancement)
- Leaflet (knowledge enhancement, attitude change)
- Diaries about complaints and diet (enhancing patients' sense of control and self-responsibility)

Laboratories
- Feedback on test requesting behaviour (knowledge enhancement)
- Small group quality improvement in local GP groups by using feedback data (social influence)

Regional cooperation of professional societies
- Problem-based laboratory test requesting forms (change of routines)

National College of General Practitioners
- Evidence-based national guidelines (knowledge enhancement, improvement of credibility of message)
- Provision of postgraduate education (knowledge enhancement)

designer – linking problem analysis, programme design and pretest and specifying the programme design phase – has yet been provided. Bartholomew et al[30,31] have done interesting work on this topic in the field of health promotion, developing intervention mapping – a systematic method of linking problem analysis, programme design and evaluation and integrating theories and scientific evidence in the design process. It also visualises the "crossroads" at which choices about the route to be followed have to be made. This method may also be applicable in designing quality of healthcare improvement interventions. Designing such interventions is an iterative process in which the designers go back and forth through the steps of problem analysis, design, and pretesting. Throughout the process, information becomes available which influences previous steps or a lack of knowledge is revealed which requires additional study.

Going through the steps of such an intervention design can be difficult and time consuming. It requires study, creativity, expertise from social sciences, and close cooperation between project group members, target population, materials designers, and implementers. A pragmatic balance should be sought between collecting information and constructing the intervention. However, since interventions are often not very effective, the investment in carefully preparing, designing, and testing such an intervention may be worthwhile.

It is important to involve future users of the intervention in the design process from the start. Writing an evaluation plan is easy after proceeding through the previous steps. As all goals have been formulated in measurable entities, measures for evaluation follow directly from the problem analysis and matrices. Besides, choices of barriers and facilitators, theories and formats have been explained so that the effects of the intervention can be linked to these in the process evaluation. The choices made might explain unexpected effects and, in the meantime, offer ideas for adjusting the intervention.

The selection criteria used during the intervention design process for barriers and facilitators, methods, strategies, formats, and materials, for example, are still mainly pragmatic and several methods are mainly theory based so further empirical research is needed to develop more evidence-based selection criteria and to test promising theories in practice. However, the systematic approach makes the intervention transparent.

We conclude that there are possibilities for designing quality improvement interventions systematically. Intervention mapping appears to be a useful method, not only for health education interventions but also for quality improvement interventions.

Key messagess

- A scientific approach is needed to the design of quality improvement interventions.
- Systematic development of interventions, including tailoring their content and format to the specific features of target groups and setting, is necessary to improve the quality of patient care.
- Decisions made during the design process are an appropriate starting point for systematic evaluations of quality improvement interventions.
- Further empirical research is needed to develop more evidence-based criteria for the selection of barriers, facilitators, theories, and strategies and to test promising theories in practice.

References

1 Bero LA, Grilli R, Grimshaw JM, *et al.* Closing the gap between research and practice: an overview of systematic reviews of interventions to promote the implementation of research findings. *BMJ* 1998;**317**:465–8.
2 Grimshaw JM, Shirran L, Thomas R, *et al.* Changing provider behaviour: an overview of systematic reviews of interventions. *Med Care* 2001;**39**(suppl 2):II2–45.
3 Campbell M, Fitzpatrick R, Haines A, *et al.* Framework for design and evaluation of complex interventions to improve health. *BMJ* 2000; **321**(suppl 2): 694–6.
4 Davis DA, Thomson MA, Oxman AD, *et al.* Changing physician performance. A systematic review of the effect of continuing medical education strategies. *JAMA* 1995;**274**:700–5.
5 Wensing M, van der Weijden T, Grol R. Implementing guidelines and innovations in general practice: which interventions are effective? *Br J Gen Pract* 1998;**48**:991–7.
6 Grol R. Beliefs and evidence in changing clinical practice. *BMJ* 1997;**315**: 418–21.
7 Grol RPTM. Implementing guidelines in general practice care. *Qual Health Care* 1992;**1**:184–91.
8 Øvretveit J. A team quality improvement sequence for complex health problems. *Qual Health Care* 1999;**8**:239–46.
9 Langley GJ, Nolan KM, Norman CL, Provost LP, Nolan TW. *The improvement guide*. San Francisco: Jossey-Bass, 1996.
10 Rogers EM. *Diffusion of innovations*. 4th ed. New York: Free Press, 1995.
11 Prochaska JO, Di Clemente CC. *The transtheoretical approach: crossing traditional boundaries of therapy*. Homewood, IL: Dow Jones-Irwin, 1984.
12 Nelson EC, Splaine ME, Batalden PB, *et al.* Building measurement and data collection into medical practice. *Ann Intern Med* 1998;**128**: 460–6.
13 Woolf SH. Practice guidelines, a new reality in medicine. II. Methods of developing guidelines. *Arch Intern Med* 1992;**152**:946–52.
14 Grimshaw JM, Eccles M, Russel I. Developing clinically valid practice guidelines. *J Eval Clin Pract* 1995;**1**:37–48.

15 Green LW, Kreuter MW. *Health promotion planning. An educational and environmental approach.* 2nd ed. Mountain View: Mayfield, 1999.
16 Kok GJ, De Vries H, Mudde AN, *et al.* Planned health education and the role of self-efficacy: Dutch research. *Health Educ Res* 1991;**6**:231–8.
17 Goodman RM, Steckler A, Kegler MC. Mobilizing organizations for health enhancement: theories of organizational change. In: Glanz K, Lewis FM, Rimer BK, eds. *Health behavior and health education: theory, research and practice.* 2nd ed. San Fransisco: Jossey-Bass, 1997:287–312.
18 Fawcett SB, Paine-Andrews A, Francisco VT, *et al.* Using empowerment theory in collaborative partnerships for community health and development. *Am J Community Psychol* 1995;**23**:677–97.
19 Minkler M, Wallerstein N. Improving health through community organization and community building. In: Glanz K, Lewis FM, Rimer BK, eds. *Health behavior and health education: theory, research and practice.* 2nd ed. San Fransisco: Jossey-Bass, 1997:241–69.
20 Cobb RW, Elder CD. *Participation in American politics: the dynamics of agenda building.* Baltimore: Johns Hopkins University Press, 1983.
21 Laumann EO, Knoke D. *The organizational state: social choice in national policy domains.* Madison: University of Wisconsin Press, 1987.
22 Pope C, Van Royen P, Baker R. Qualitative methods in research on healthcare quality. *Qual Saf Health Care* 2002;**11**:148–52.
23 Fishbein M, Ajzen I. *Belief, attitude, intention and behavior: an introduction to theory and research.* Reading, MA: Addison Wesley, 1975.
24 McGuire WJ. Attitudes and attitude change. In: Lindzey G, Aronson E, eds. *The handbook of social psychology.* New York: Random House, 1985: 233–346.
25 Miles MB, Huberman AM. *Qualitative data analysis. An expanded sourcebook.* Thousand Oaks: Sage, 1994.
26 Zaat JO, Van Eijk JT, Bonte HA. Laboratory test form design influences test ordering by general practitioners in the Netherlands. *Med Care* 1992;**30**:189–98.
27 Winkens RAG. *Improving test ordering in general practice. The effects of individual feedback.* Rijksuniversiteit Limburg, 1994.
28 van der Weijden T, van Velsen M, Dinant GJ, *et al.* Unexplained complaints in general practice. Prevalence, patient expectations, and the professional's test ordering behavior. *Med Decision Making* 2003;**23**:226–31.
29 van der Weijden T, van Bokhoven MA, Dinant GJ, *et al.* Understanding laboratory testing in diagnostic uncertainty: a qualitative study in general practice. *Br J Gen Pract* 2002;**52**:974–80.
30 Bartholomew LK, Parcel GS, Kok G. Intervention mapping: a process for developing theory- and evidence-based health education programs. *Health Educ Behav* 1998;**25**:545–63.
31 Bartholomew LK, Parcel GS, Kok G, Gottlieb NH. *Intervention mapping. Designing theory- and evidence-based health promotion programs.* Mountain View: Mayfield, 2001.
32 Marlatt GA, Gordon JR. *Relapse prevention: maintenance strategies in the treatment of addictive behaviors.* New York: Guilford, 1985.
33 Bero L, Grilli R, Grimshaw JM, *et al.* Cochrane Effective Practice and Organisation of Care Group. *Cochrane Library.* Issue 3. Oxford: Update Software, 2002.
34 Glanz K, Lewis FM, Rimer BK. *Health behavior and health education: theory, research and practice.* 2nd ed. San Francisco: Jossey-Bass, 1997.

11: Process evaluation of quality improvement interventions

MARLIES HULSCHER, MIRANDA LAURANT,
RICHARD GROL

To design potentially successful quality improvement (QI) interventions, it is crucial to make use of detailed breakdowns of the implementation processes of successful and unsuccessful interventions. Process evaluation can throw light on the mechanisms responsible for the result obtained in the intervention group. It enables researchers and implementers to (1) describe the intervention in detail, (2) check actual exposure to the intervention, and (3) describe the experience of those exposed. This chapter presents a framework containing features of QI interventions that might influence success. Attention is paid to features of the target group, the implementers or change agents, the frequency of intervention activities, and features of the information imparted. The framework can be used as a starting point to address all three aspects of process evaluation mentioned above. Process evaluation can be applied to small scale improvement projects, controlled QI studies, and large scale QI programmes; in each case it plays a different role.

A wide variety of quality improvement (QI) interventions can be used in health care. Reviews show that most interventions are effective in some settings but not in others.[1–3] Studies of effective intervention programmes have shown varying and often modest improvements in healthcare performance. To understand in more detail why some interventions are successful while others fail to change practice, it is necessary to gain insight into the "black box" of QI interventions. Studying the black box of (un)successful interventions implies that we

Box 11.1 Why is it important to look inside the "black box" of the intervention?

Szczepura et al[4] concluded that an intervention involving feedback failed to change professional practice, whereas Nattinger et al[5] showed that feedback led to significant improvements in professional care. However, careful analysis of the feedback applied in these studies showed that the QI interventions had different characters.

In the study by Szczepura et al general practitioners (GPs) in the intervention group received three sets of information about the care they had provided – at the start, after 12 months, and after 24 months. This information concerned cervical cancer screening, developmental screening/immunisation in children, and the determination of risk factors in persons aged 35–64 years such as blood pressure, alcohol consumption, smoking, and body weight. GPs in the so-called "graphic" feedback group received a profile containing the following values for each feedback item: group minimum, group maximum, median, and 20th and 80th percentiles; at each practice the GPs' own scores were marked clearly. The GPs in the control group received feedback in table form – that is, an overview of their own values accompanied by the minimum and maximum scores in the total group. Neither intervention was effective. On receipt of the comparative feedback information all GPs were asked to rate the feedback in terms of its acceptability and intelligibility and whether or not regular feedback in this form was helpful to the practice. No differences regarding these items were reported. No information was provided by the authors on actual exposure of the target population to the intervention – for example, how many actually read the feedback report.

In the study by Nattinger et al, performed over a period of 6 months, general internists received monthly overviews of the percentage of patients who had been treated in accordance with the mammography guideline. The first 3 months concerned only the individual management of the internist in question, whereas the second 3 months concerned individual management compared with the management of an anonymous group of colleagues presented with the aid of a histogram. This feedback proved to be effective. The authors stated that they were unable to say how many physicians had actually read their feedback. Thus, no information was provided on actual exposure or the experience of those exposed.

can no longer confine ourselves to describing a QI intervention in global terms – for example, merely as "feedback", "reminders", or "a combination of a CME seminar, free office materials, and one office visit by a staff member" (Box 11.1). The concrete activities taken as part of the QI intervention, the actual exposure of participants to these activities, together with their experience of these activities, may influence the final result (success or failure). Process evaluation can throw light on the mechanisms and processes responsible for the result and the variation in results in the target group.

Process evaluation is an important tool that can meticulously describe the QI intervention itself, the actual exposure to this intervention, and the experience of those exposed (participants) (Box 11.2). This information is not only crucial for understanding the success – or lack of success – of QI interventions, but also for providing basic data for economic evaluation of quality improvement. Although the latter is beyond the scope of this review, it enables estimates to be made of the cost in terms of time and/or money (see Chapter 13).

This chapter explores the purpose and value of process evaluation of QI interventions and addresses the issue of what data should be collected ("what to measure") and data collection methods ("how to measure").

Box 11.2 Process evaluation

Process evaluation can be used:

(1) to describe the QI intervention – for example:

- What was the exact nature of the QI intervention?
- What material investments, time investments, etc were required?

(2) To check the actual exposure to the QI intervention – for example:

- Was the QI intervention implemented according to plan?
- Was the target population actually exposed to the intervention as planned?
- Does this offer an explanation for not achieving the goals?

(3) To describe the experience of those exposed to the QI intervention – for example:

- How did the target group experience the intervention and the changes?
- What problems arose while implementing the changes?
- What requirements for change were experienced?

Purpose and value of process evaluation

The results of process evaluation serve different purposes.

- A description of the "intervention as planned" acts as a blueprint to help change agents (and researchers) to apply the intervention as intended in a uniform way within the target population.
- Actual exposure can be established by checking whether the intervention was performed as planned. This information can be used to adapt the intervention if necessary. Researchers or evaluators can use the information later to explain success or lack of effect, particularly when they do not want to change the intervention during the course of a study. If the intervention in its ultimate form differs considerably from the original plan, then this can be put down to "implementation error".[6] Failing to detect differences between the original intervention plan and the ultimate manner of implementation is sometimes referred to as a "type III error" (an analogy with the statistical type I and type II errors).[6]
- A blueprint of the "intervention as performed" is important to enable other people to replicate the intervention. In addition, a detailed description of the "intervention as performed" will facilitate future comparisons between studies and (meta) analysis of crucial features of effective interventions.
- The main purpose of gaining detailed insight into the experience of those exposed to the intervention is to revise the QI intervention in question. This information on influencing factors as experienced by participants can be used to improve the intervention either during its application (the developmental approach) or afterwards (the experimental approach).

Process evaluation and quality improvement interventions: examples

Process evaluation can be applied to QI interventions at any stage of their development. Here we distinguish between QI interventions at three stages of development: (1) pilot studies or small scale improvement projects, (2) controlled QI studies, and (3) large scale QI programmes. Process evaluation plays a different role in each case.

Pilot studies/small scale improvement projects

Effect evaluation of a newly developed QI intervention that is being tested in a pilot study or used within a small scale improvement project yields an estimate of the potential level of change. Process evaluation can provide important answers to questions on the feasibility and applicability of introducing the intervention; such answers might prompt revision of the improvement activities in the intervention. Thus, researchers and implementers of this type of QI intervention can use process information to investigate whether they are on the right track or whether their approach needs adjustment.

Controlled QI studies

In a controlled study of the effectiveness of a QI intervention, the central issue is testing the effectiveness of the implementation method in standardised circumstances. In this case, process evaluation yields information that can help to explain heterogeneity in effects. Process evaluation is important to check whether the planned improvement activities have indeed been executed in a uniform way and whether the target population has actually been exposed to these activities as planned. Researchers and implementers of these QI interventions can use process information to detect gaps in implementation that might be responsible for failure or the disappointing outcome of an intervention. Another use for process evaluation in such studies is to determine how the participants experienced the activities: whether they encountered any bottlenecks while implementing the changes and whether they were satisfied with the intervention method. Together with data on the implementation of the QI intervention, this might explain why some participants successfully improved the quality of care while others did not, or why some participants were more successful than others (see example in Box 11.3).

Box 11.3 Improving the prevention of cardiovascular disease[7]

The study investigated the effectiveness of and experience with an, at that time, innovative method of introducing guidelines to improve the organisation of preventive activities in general practice. Over a period of 18 months, trained outreach visitors spent time solving problems in the organisation of prevention in general practice. The study showed that guidelines to organise prevention of cardiovascular disease in general practice could be introduced effectively (controlled study). To evaluate the scope and limitations of the QI intervention, process information was gathered at the end of the project from all the participants at the intervention practices (68 GPs and 83 practice assistants at 33 general practices). Information was collected on actual exposure to the QI intervention, experience with the intervention in general and with the outreach visitors, bottlenecks and advantages, results of the intervention regarding the number of newly detected patients at risk, and the influence of the intervention on the working methods of the GPs and practice assistants.

During 18 months of the intervention the practices were visited between 13 and 59 times (mean 25, SD 9). The mean duration of a visit was 73 minutes (SD 43) with a minimum of 0 minutes (delivering materials only) and a maximum of almost 5 hours. Practices spent, on average, 45% of the visit hours on training and 52% on conferring. The number of team members with whom the outreach visitors met ranged from 1 to 14. In 63% of the consultations the outreach visitor met with practice assistants only, in 7% she met with GPs only, and in 30% of the cases she met both practice assistants and GPs.

In 27 of the practices, adherence to guidelines increased for at least three guidelines, leading to a mean final adherence score of eight guidelines (minimum 7, maximum 9). These practices were visited on average 25 times for almost 31 hours. In five practices no increase or only a very small increase in adherence to guidelines was shown, leading to a mean final adherence score of four guidelines. In these practices the average number of visits (20) and the total duration of the visits (19 hours) were below the group average.

The majority of GPs and practice assistants had a positive opinion of the QI intervention. They were satisfied about the outreach visits, but the practice assistants experienced extra workload due to the QI intervention. Practice assistants expressed more complaints about the paperwork involved than the GPs, but mentioned fewer patient barriers. Practice assistants and, to a smaller extent, GPs remarked that their participation in the intervention had improved their work methods. Relationships were found between the experience of the participants and the degree to which the practice had changed: more positive experiences of the participants about the QI intervention in general and more newly detected patients than expected were related to more change.

Box 11.4 Cervical cancer screening[8]

In a national prevention programme GPs and practice assistants were exposed, over a period of 2·5 years, to a combined strategy to introduce guidelines for cervical cancer screening. The combination comprised formulating and distributing guidelines, supplying educative material and a software module, and providing financial support on a national level. On a regional level, agreements were made between the relevant parties (GPs, municipal health services, comprehensive cancer centres, pathology laboratories), and continuing medical education (CME) meetings were organised for GPs and practice assistants. On a local level, trained outreach visitors called at the practices. The evaluation (in a random one-in-three sample, response 62%, 988 practices) showed considerable improvements at the practices: after the intervention adherence to 9 of the 10 key indicators had been improved. Information on actual exposure to programme elements was collected by postal questionnaire. Almost all practices in the study population (94%) had been informed about the national prevention programme. For practices that had had contact with an outreach visitor through a practice visit (40%), the median number of practice visits was 2 (range 1–13). The software modules were used by 474 practices (48%), either in full or in part.

Crucial elements for the successful implementation of the guidelines were:

- making use of the software module (odds ratios (ORs) 1·85–10·2 for nine indicators);
- having received two or more outreach visits (ORs 1·46–2·35 for six indicators); and
- practice assistants having attended the refresher course (ORs 1·37–1·90 for four indicators).

Large scale QI programmes

In a large scale QI programme effectiveness analyses can show the extent to which the goals of the intervention have been achieved, whereas process evaluation provides information about the actual intervention and about exposure to and experience with the intervention. In case a control group is lacking, the results of process evaluation might yield information about the relationship between the QI intervention and the changes achieved (see example in Box 11.4).

What to measure

If it is decided to perform a process evaluation, researchers and implementers of QI interventions are faced with the following questions:

- What "key features" of the QI intervention should be included in the description (before and/or after intervention) because they might cause or influence the effect of the intervention? This is the main question for those interested in developing a blueprint of the intervention, (a) to support uniform performance of the intervention, (b) to enable replication of the intervention, or (c) to facilitate comparisons and meta-analysis of QI interventions.
- What features of the QI intervention are important to measure (or monitor) while checking whether the participants were exposed as planned? This is the main question for those interested in (a) adapting the QI intervention during the course of the intervention or (b) explaining success or lack of success afterwards.
- What are "crucial success and failure factors" as experienced by those exposed that might cause or influence the effect of the QI intervention? This is the main question for people interested in revising the QI intervention in question.

To provide practical guidance to researchers and implementers of QI interventions, we present some of our work that addressed these questions in process evaluation of QI interventions. The framework shown here can be used as a starting point in answering all three types of questions.

What to measure: a framework

On the basis of several theories that underlie different approaches to changing clinical practice,[9–13] we developed a framework containing features of QI interventions that might influence their success or failure. We also used the checklist developed by the Cochrane Effective Practice and Organisation of Care Review Group (EPOC)[14] to guide reviewers when extracting relevant information from primary studies. In addition, we used a number of reviews on the effectiveness of various interventions[2] and explored the literature on process and programme evaluation.[6,15–20]

The resulting framework was tested on a convenience sample of 29 published studies that had used different QI interventions.[21] We approached the 26 authors of these studies (response rate 86%). Many features of the intervention were not adequately described in the publications or were not described at all, but most authors were able to provide the lacking information when asked. The framework was revised based on the results of this pilot study.

In the framework (Table 11.1) attention is paid to features of the target group, the implementers or change agents, the frequency of intervention activities, and the features of the information imparted. The left column gives a general description of the feature of an intervention that is described in more detail in the right column.

How to measure

What methods (single or combined) can be used to gather process data?

Depending on the main question being addressed by process evaluation, it is possible to take a more developmental approach (qualitative and inductive, see also Chapter 4) or a more experimental approach (quantitative and deductive). Information can be gathered by on-site observation (on the spot or audio/video recording), from self-reports (interviews and questionnaires or surveys), and from existing data sources (or secondary sources). Examples of secondary sources include minutes of meetings, bills, purchase orders, invoices, end of chapter tests, certificates upon completion of activities, attendance logs, signing in and signing out sheets, checklists, referral letters, diaries, news releases, etc.[6,15–20]

When choosing a measurement method (or a series of methods), it is important to consider the existing circumstances (for example, the amount of time available for gathering and interpreting data), practical issues, the homogeneity of the data, privacy and confidentiality, and the estimated tolerance levels of the respondents who will be asked to provide data. In

Table 11.1 Framework for describing the key features of a QI intervention

Relevant features of the intervention	How to elicit the information
1 Global typing of the intervention (see also the EPOC checklist)	• Describe the type of intervention concerned • Interventions orientated towards health professionals, e.g. (a) distribution of educational materials (b) patient mediated interventions (c) etc • Organisational interventions, e.g. (a) provider orientated interventions: (i) revision of professional roles (ii) etc (b) patient orientated interventions: (i) mail order pharmacies (ii) etc (c) structural interventions: (i) changes to the setting/site of service delivery (ii) etc • Financial interventions, e.g. (a) care-provider financial interventions: (i) fee for service (ii) etc (b) patient financial interventions: (i) co-payment (ii) etc • Regulatory interventions, e.g. (a) management of patient complaints (b) etc
If multiple options have been mentioned above, then the features of each of the options must be filled in separately	
2 Target group/participants	
2.1 Professional status or patient categories	• Describe the professions of the participants or the patient categories that the intervention is aimed at
2.2 Interaction between participants	• Describe whether the intervention is aimed at individuals or members of a group • If the intervention is aimed at group members, describe whether the group is homogeneous or heterogeneous

(Continued)

Table 11.1 (*Continued*)

Relevant features of the intervention	How to elicit the information
2.3 Size of the target group	• Describe the total number of groups that the intervention is aimed at • Describe the size of each group • Describe the number of individuals per profession or patient category (these may be members of a number of groups) that the intervention is aimed at (e.g. 70 internists and 110 diabetic nurses)
2.4 Motivation for participation	• Describe the motivation behind participation (e.g. voluntary or obligatory participation, accreditation, financial reward, etc)
3 Implementer	
3.1 Professional status	• Describe the professional backgrounds of the implementers, i.e. the individuals who have actual contact with the target group (the instructor, the feedback provider, etc)
3.2 Opinion leaders	• Describe whether the individual who implements the intervention can be considered as opinion leader for the target group
3.3 Authority	• Describe the authority on whose basis the intervention is implemented (e.g. the implementer is an expert, representative for the target group, has power, etc)
4 Frequency	
4.1 Number	• Describe the number of identical intervention activities (e.g. sending feedback reports on 4 occasions, making 5 visits to the practice, organising 1 CME meeting)
4.2 Time intervals	• Describe the time intervals between the above mentioned identical intervention activities
4.3 Duration	• Describe the duration of each identical intervention activity at each contact meeting

(Continued)

Table 11.1 (*Continued*)

Relevant features of the intervention	How to elicit the information
5 Information about the innovation	
5.1 Type of information about the innovation or guideline	• Describe the type of information that was given in the intervention about the innovation (e.g. the actual text of a published guideline, information on certain recommendations or indicators)
5.2 Presentation form of the information about the innovation or guideline	• Describe the presentation form of the information provided (e.g. descriptive, illustrative, graphic, tables, etc)
5.3 Medium	• Describe how the information was provided (e.g. verbally, written, automated, etc)
6 Information about target group management/performance	
6.1 Type of information about performance	• Describe the type of information that was given in the intervention about the performance of the target group (e.g. information about individual performance regarding certain patient categories, information about the performance of the total group of participants, information about individual performance as measured with paper cases, information about national reference values, etc)
6.2 Presentation form of the information about performance	• Describe the presentation form of the information provided (e.g. descriptive, illustrative, graphic, tables, etc)
6.3 Medium	• Describe how the information was provided (e.g. verbally, written, automated, etc)
6.4 Feasibility of comparing information on performance	• Describe the feasibility of comparing individual performance with that of others or with general criteria (guidelines, recommendations)

addition, the instruments must be simple and user friendly so that they are not burdensome for the user. On the other hand, they must be detailed enough to answer the evaluation questions and goals. When selecting the instruments, it is necessary to consider whether the method of data gathering will have an undesirable influence on the ongoing investigation or intervention implementation, depending on the study design or type of project. It must also be guaranteed that the data will be gathered in a valid and reliable manner from selected population samples. Depending on the approach taken (developmental or experimental), respondent samples can be selected to reflect the diversity within a given population (purposive sampling) or to achieve statistical representativeness. Whatever method is chosen, the persons responsible for data gathering should have received adequate training in the skills and terms associated with the use of the instruments and be able to perform quality control checks.

Describing the QI intervention

How do we elicit the information to describe the "intervention as planned" or the "intervention as performed"?

The implementers or researchers can be asked to fill in the framework to describe the features of the QI intervention as planned before starting the intervention. Interviews with the programme developers and associated parties can provide information. As a basis, it may be useful to fall back on existing documentation such as the study plan, the programme proposal, minutes of meetings, or existing records.

To describe the QI intervention as performed (after its implementation), use can be made of interviews with the implementers of the intervention and/or the participants, or questionnaires and surveys. Participants can often provide useful information about the intervention as performed in terms of their personal participation during implementation. However, the reliability of data reported in retrospect decreases as the complexity and extensiveness of the intervention increases, and as the interval since start of the intervention increases and it becomes longer ago that the persons were exposed to intervention activities. Moreover, the framework involves a great many features and details that the respondents may not have been aware of during the intervention, which once again makes it difficult to obtain valid data after the event. It is therefore often preferable to gather information during the process and to use these data to describe the intervention in its ultimate form (see below).

Checking actual exposure to the QI intervention

How can we measure actual exposure to the QI intervention?

The implementation of intervention activities can be studied periodically, continuously, or retrospectively by obtaining information from the respondents (implementers or participants), by using observation, self-reports and/or existing data sources. If possible, information should be gathered on all the features. However, it is no small task to verify whether the participants are performing the intended intervention activities. Because of resource restraints, for example, it may be necessary to select several central features of the intervention and pay the closest attention to them. During the implementation of QI interventions, sometimes it is permitted (and sometimes it is not permitted) for the execution process to vary across sites or across time. When checking exposure, the following rule of thumb can be used: the greater the variation allowed, the more attention must be paid to the feature concerned. The remaining features could then be measured by one simple method (see example in Box 11.5).

Describing the experience of those exposed to the QI intervention

How can data be gathered on the experience of persons exposed to the QI intervention?

Participants can be asked, during and/or after the intervention, to provide self-reported information on how they experienced the QI intervention, including whether they perceived factors related to success or failure. Thus, opinions can be explored on the type(s) of intervention chosen and on all features of each type of intervention. Participants can also

Box 11.5 Improving the prevention of cardiovascular disease[7]

The multifaceted intervention as planned consisted of four types of intervention:

(1) Providing all practice members with information about the guidelines and project. The information was provided by the outreach visitor during an introductory visit (standardised with the help of a checklist).
(2) Providing feedback on current practice. After an analysis of the practice organisation (standardised with the help of checklists), all practice members received a feedback report on current practice regarding all guidelines.
(3) Tailoring outreach visits from trained nurses. After receiving the feedback report, the practice members chose and discussed intended changes under the guidance of an outreach visitor. The outreach visitor helped the practice to implement the changes. Outreach visits were arranged according to needs and wishes.
(4) Tailoring the provision of educational materials and practical tools. Depending on their needs and wishes, practice members were provided with standardised educational materials and tools.

It was decided – mainly for practical reasons such as time and money constraints – that it would be most valuable to monitor the tailoring activities of the intervention – that is, the outreach visits and the materials received by the practice team (in which variation was allowed). In addition, the researchers repeatedly stressed the importance of using the checklists and determined the timing and content of the feedback.

To check actual exposure to the outreach visits and materials, a simple coded visit registration form was developed (and pilot tested) that had to be filled in by the outreach visitor after each visit to a practice. The following features of a visit had to be recorded:

- the date and duration of the visit;
- the participants in a meeting (name and function);
- the type of activities during a meeting; and
- the materials used or provided during a meeting.

Box 11.3 describes how this information was ultimately used by the researchers to describe the intervention as performed.

describe features they perceived as being most related to the outcome of the intervention (success or failure). In this way, information is obtained that is closely and directly linked to the intervention method as experienced (see example in Box 11.6).

Box 11.6 Process evaluation of a tailored multifaceted approach to changing general practice care patterns and improving preventive care[22]

Prevention facilitators (outreach visitors) tailored the following strategies to the needs and unique circumstances of 22 general practices (54 GPs):

- audit and ongoing feedback;
- consensus building;
- opinion leaders and networking;
- academic detailing and education materials;
- reminder systems;
- patient mediated activities;
- patient education materials.

Effect evaluation showed an absolute improvement over time of 11·5% in preventive care performance (13 preventive strategies, e.g. counselling for folic acid, advice to quit smoking, influenza vaccination, glucose testing, PSA testing).

The aim of process evaluation was to document the extent of conformity with the QI intervention during implementation and to gain insight into why the intervention successfully improved preventive care. Key measures in the evaluation process were the frequency of delivery of the intervention components (i.e. the different types of intervention), the time involved, the scope of delivery, the utility of the components, and GP satisfaction with the intervention.

Five data collection tools were used, as well as a combination of descriptive, quantitative, and qualitative analyses. Triangulation was employed to investigate the quality of the implementation activities.

The facilitator documented her activities and progress on two structured forms known as the weekly activity sheet (hours spent on on-site and off-site activities) and the monthly narrative report (per practice: number of visits; activities and their outcomes; number of participants; plan for the following month). At 6 months and 17 months two GP members of the research team conducted semi-structured telephone interviews with the participating GPs to find out whether they were happy or unhappy with the interventions and to document their ideas about improvement and overall satisfaction (close ended questions). Facilitators interviewed contact practitioners to obtain post-intervention feedback about their experience. GPs were sent a questionnaire by mail to report any changes that had taken place over the preceding 18 months.

Facilitators generally visited the practices to deliver the audit and feedback, consensus building, and reminder system components. All the study practices received preventive performance audit and feedback, achieved consensus on a plan for improvement, and

(Continued)

Box 11.6 *(Continued)*

implemented a reminder system. 90% of the practices implemented a customised flow sheet while 10% used a computerised reminder system; 95% of the intervention practices wanted evidence for prevention, 82% participated in a workshop, and 100% received patient education material in a binder.

Content analysis of the data obtained during the GP interviews and bivariate analysis of GP self-reported changes compared with a non-intervention control group of GPs revealed that audit and feedback, consensus building, and development of reminder systems were the key intervention components.

Analysing barriers and facilitators while participating in the intervention and implementing the changes can also provide useful insights into how the QI intervention might be revised. The framework presented in Table 11.1 does not provide help with this aspect of process evaluation. Ideally, a QI intervention that aims to change clinical practice is designed on the basis of a systematic scientific approach that (a) analyses barriers and facilitators and (b) links the intervention to these influencing factors (see also Chapters 4 and 10). A complete analysis of the experience of participants, with the aim of gaining insight into how the QI intervention might be revised, should therefore also check whether barriers and facilitators were indeed successfully handled.

Conclusions

Process evaluation performed in a pilot study or small scale improvement project, a controlled QI study, or a large scale QI programme can throw light on the mechanisms and processes responsible for the result in the target group. In this way, process evaluation makes a very relevant and desirable contribution to the development of potentially successful QI interventions. The framework presented here gives the key features necessary to describe a QI intervention in detail, to check whether the intervention was performed as planned, and to assess the experience of participants.

Key messages

- To understand why some QI interventions successfully bring about improvement while others fail to change practice, it is necessary to look into the "black box" of interventions and study the determinants of success or failure.
- Process evaluation contributes significantly to the development of potentially successful QI interventions.
- Process evaluation helps to describe the QI intervention itself, the actual exposure to the intervention, and the experience of the people exposed.
- A framework is presented in which attention is paid to features of the target group, the implementers or change agents, the frequency of intervention activities, and the features of the information imparted. All of these features might influence the success of the QI intervention in question.
- Process evaluation is an intensive task that requires great attention to detail.

References

1 Anon. Getting evidence into practice. *Effective Health Care* 1999;**5**:1–15.
2 Bero L, Grilli R, Grimshaw JM, *et al*. Closing the gap between research and practice: an overview of systematic reviews of interventions to promote implementation of research findings by health care professionals. *BMJ* 1998;**317**:465–8.
3 Grol R. Beliefs and evidence in changing clinical practice. *BMJ* 1997;**315**:418–21.
4 Szczepura A, Wilmot J, Davies C, *et al*. Effectiveness and cost of different strategies for information feedback in general practice. *Br J Gen Pract* 1994;**43**:19–24.
5 Nattinger AB, Panzer RJ, Janus J. Improving the utilization of screening mammography in primary care practices. *Arch Intern Med* 1989;**149**:2087–92.
6 Swanborn PG. *Evaluation. The design, support and evaluation of interventions: a methodological basis for evaluation research* (in Dutch). Amsterdam: Uitgeverij Boom, 1999.
7 Hulscher MEJL, van Drenth BB, Mokkink HGA, *et al*. Tailored outreach visits as a method for implementing guidelines and improving preventive care. *Int J Qual Health Care* 1998;**10**:105–12.
8 Hermens RPMG, Hak E, Hulscher MEJL, *et al*. Adherence to guidelines on cervical cancer screening in general practice: programme elements of successful implementation. *Br J Gen Pract* 2001;**51**:897–903.
9 McGuire WJ. Attitudes and attitude change. In: Lindzey G, Aronson E. *The handbook of social psychology.* 3rd ed. New York: Random House, 1985: 233–346.
10 Ajzen I. The theory of planned behaviour. *Organ Behav Hum Decis Process* 1991;**50**:179–211.
11 Bandura A. *Social foundations of thought and action: a social cognitive theory.* New York: Prentice-Hall, 1986.

12 Festinger L. A theory of social comparison processes. *Human Relations* 1954;7:117–40.
13 Rogers EM. *Diffusion of innovations*. New York: The Free Press, 1983.
14 Cochrane Effective Practice and Organisation of Care Review Group (EPOC). *The data collection checklist*. 1998.
15 King JA, Morris LL, Fitz-Gibbon CT. How to assess program implementation. In: Herman JL, ed. *Program evaluation kit*. Newbury Park, CA: Sage, 1987.
16 Herman JL, Morris LL, Fitz-Gibbon CT. Evaluator's Handbook. In: Herman JL, ed. *Program evaluation kit*. Newbury Park, CA: Sage, 1987.
17 Fink A. *Evaluation fundamentals guiding health programs, research, and policy*. Newbury Park, CA: Sage Publications, 1993.
18 Rossi PH, Freeman HE. *Evaluation: a systematic approach*. Newbury Park, CA: Sage, 1993.
19 Rossi PH, Freeman HE, Lipsey MW. *Evaluation. A systematic approach*. Thousand Oaks, CA: Sage, 1999.
20 Øvretveit J. *Evaluating health interventions: an introduction to evaluation of health treatments, services, policies and organizational interventions*. Buckingham: Open University Press, 2000.
21 Laurant M, Hulscher M, Wensing M, *et al*. *Analysing and monitoring implementation strategies for changing professional practice*. Nijmegen: WOK, 1999.
22 Baskerville NB, Hogg W, Lemelin J. Process evaluation of a tailored multifaceted approach to changing family physician practice patterns and improving preventive care. *J Fam Pract* 2001;**50**:W242–9.

12: Statistical process control as a tool for research and healthcare improvement

JAMES C BENNEYAN, ROBERT C LLOYD,
PAUL E PLSEK

Improvement of health care requires making changes in processes of care and service delivery. Although process performance is measured to determine if these changes are having the desired beneficial effects, this analysis is complicated by the existence of natural variation – that is, repeated measurements naturally yield different values and, even if nothing was done, a subsequent measurement might seem to indicate a better or worse performance. Traditional statistical analysis methods account for natural variation but require aggregation of measurements over time, which can delay decision making. Statistical process control (SPC) is a branch of statistics that combines rigorous time series analysis methods with graphical presentation of data, often yielding insights into the data more quickly and in a way more understandable to lay decision makers. SPC and its primary tool – the control chart – provide researchers and practitioners with a method of better understanding and communicating data from healthcare improvement efforts. This paper provides an overview of SPC and several practical examples of healthcare applications of control charts.

All improvement requires change, but not all change results in improvement.[1] The key to identifying beneficial change is measurement. The major components of measurement include: (1) determining and defining key indicators; (2) collecting an appropriate amount of data; and (3) analysing and interpreting these data. This chapter focuses on the third component – the analysis and interpretation of data – using statistical process control (SPC). SPC charts can help both researchers and practitioners of quality improvement to determine whether changes in processes are making a real difference in outcomes. We describe the problem that variation poses in analysis, give an overview of statistical process control theory, explain control charts (a major tool of SPC), and provide examples of their application to common issues in healthcare improvement.

Variation in measurement

Interpretation of data to detect change is not always a simple matter. Repeated measures of the same parameter often yield slightly different results – for example, re-measurement of a patient's blood pressure, a department's waiting times, or appointment access satisfaction – even if there is no fundamental change. This inherent variability is due to factors such as fluctuations in patients' biological processes, differences in service processes, and imperfections in the measurement process itself.

How large a fluctuation in the data must be observed in order to be reasonably sure that an improvement has actually occurred? Like other statistical methods, SPC helps to tease out the variability inherent within any process so that both researchers and practitioners of quality improvement can better understand whether interventions have had the desired impact and, if so, whether the improvement is sustainable beyond the time period under study.

The researcher designs formal studies in which data are collected at different points in time or place for comparison, such as a randomised clinical trial to evaluate the impact of a new cholesterol lowering drug. In this type of study the goal may be to test the null hypothesis that there is no difference between an experimental group and a control group who did not receive the drug. Many formal research designs exist to handle the numerous possible variations of such studies,[2] including double blind randomised clinical trials.

At the other end of the spectrum, the improvement practitioner often takes a simpler approach to research designs. This person may be interested in comparing the performance of a process at one site with itself – for example, looking at data collected before and after a change has been introduced – or in contrasting the performance of two or more sites over time. However, both the researcher and the practitioner essentially end up addressing the same question – namely, "What can be concluded from sets of measurements taken before and after the time of a change, given that these measurements would probably show some variation even if there had been no purposeful change?"

An advantage of SPC is that classical statistical methods typically are based on "time static" statistical tests with all data aggregated into large samples that ignore their time order – for example, the mean waiting time at intervention sites might be compared with that at non-intervention sites. Tests of significance are usually the statistical tool of preference used to see if one group is "significantly different" from the other. These are useful methods and have good statistical power when based on sufficiently large data sets. The delay in accumulating a sufficient amount of data, however, often limits the application of these methods in practice in health care and practitioners may resort to simple bar charts, line graphs, or tables to present the data. In this case the practitioner can only make a qualitative statement about whether or not there "seems" to be an improvement.

In contrast, SPC methods combine the rigour of classical statistical methods with the time sensitivity of pragmatic improvement. By integrating the power of statistical significance tests with chronological analysis of graphs of summary data as they are produced, SPC is able to detect process changes and trends earlier. While this may be a less familiar branch of statistics to many researchers, it is no less valid. SPC also distils statistical theory into relatively simple formulae and graphical displays that can easily be used by non-statisticians.

Theory of statistical process control

The basic theory of statistical process control was developed in the late 1920s by Dr Walter Shewhart,[3] a statistician at the AT&T Bell Laboratories in the USA, and was popularised worldwide by Dr W Edwards Deming.[4] Both observed that repeated measurements from a process will exhibit variation – Shewhart originally worked with manufacturing processes but he and Deming quickly realised that their observation could be applied to any sort of process. If a process is stable, its variation will be predictable and can be described by one of several statistical distributions.

One such model of random variation is the normal (or Gaussian) bell shaped distribution which is familiar to most healthcare professionals. While repeated measurements from many processes follow normal distributions, it is important to note that there are many other types of distributions that describe the variation in other healthcare measurements such as Poisson, binomial, or geometric distributions. For example, the random variation in the number of wound infections after surgery will follow a binomial distribution since there are only two possible outcomes – each patient either did or did not have a postoperative infection with about the same probability (assuming that the data are adjusted for patient acuity, surgical techniques, and other such variables).

SPC theory uses the phrase "common cause variation" to refer to the natural variation inherent in a process on a regular basis. This is the variation that is expected to occur according to the underlying statistical distribution if its parameters remain constant over time. For example, the random variation between body temperatures within a population of healthy people is a result of basic human physiology, while the random variation in week to week wound infection rates is a result of factors such as training, sources of supplies, surgical and nursing care practices, and cleanliness procedures. Processes that exhibit only common cause variation are said to be stable, predictable, and in "statistical control", hence the major tool of SPC is called the "statistical control chart".

Conversely, the phrase "special cause variation" refers to unnatural variation due to events, changes, or circumstances that have not previously been typical or inherent in the regular process. This is similar to the concept in traditional hypothesis tests of data exhibiting statistically significant differences, a key distinction being that we now test for changes graphically and over time using small samples. For example, heavy demand for accident and emergency (A&E) services brought on by an influenza epidemic may create special cause variation (statistically significant differences) in the form of increases in A&E waiting times. As another example, suppose that the daily mean turn around time (TAT) for a particular laboratory test is 64 minutes with a minimum of 45 minutes and a maximum of 83 minutes; this mean has been observed for several months. One day the mean jumps to 97 minutes because a major power outage caused the computers to go down, the lights to go out, and the pneumatic tube system to become inoperative. On this particular day the process is said to be "out of control" and incapable of performing as it had in the past due to the "special cause" of the power outage.

Note that special cause variation can be the result of either a deliberate intervention or an external event over which we have little control. Special causes of variation can also be transient (being short staffed in A&E one day due to illness of a key person) or can become part of the permanent common cause system (eliminating a staff position through a budget cut).

Interventions in a research study or change ideas in a quality improvement project are deliberate attempts to introduce special causes of variation. Statistical tools are therefore needed to help distinguish whether patterns in a set of measurements exhibit common or special cause variation. While statistical process control charts and hypothesis tests are both designed to achieve this goal, an important difference is that SPC provides a graphical, simpler, and often faster way to answer this question. The basic principles of SPC are summarised in Box 12.1.

These observations lead to two general approaches for improving processes. Because processes that exhibit special cause variation are unstable and unpredictable, they should be

Box 12.1 Basic principles of SPC

- Individual measurements from any process will exhibit variation.
- If the data come from a stable common cause process, their variability is predictable within a knowable range that can be computed from a statistical model such as the Gaussian, binomial, or Poisson distribution.
- If processes produce data with special causes, measured values will deviate in some observable way from these random distribution models.
- Assuming the data are in control, we can establish statistical limits and test for data that deviate from predictions, providing statistical evidence of a change.

improved by first eliminating the special causes in order to bring the process "into control". In contrast, processes that exhibit only common cause variation will continue to produce the same results, within statistical limits, unless the process is fundamentally changed or redesigned.

Moreover, if a process remains in control, future measurements will continue to follow the same probability distribution as previously – that is, if a stable process produces data that follow a normal distribution and it is not further disturbed by special causes, we can expect about 95% of future measurements to fall within ±2 standard deviations (SD) around the mean. We can make similar statements about prediction ranges associated with any other statistical distribution. In general, regardless of the underlying distribution, almost all data will fall within ±3SD of the mean if the underlying distribution is stable – that is, if the process is in statistical control.

The control chart therefore defines what the process is capable of producing given its current design and operation. If a different level of performance is wanted in the future, we must intervene and introduce a change in the process – that is, a special cause. If we simply want to sustain the current level of performance, special causes of variation must be prevented or eliminated. Control charts can often help to detect special cause variation more easily and faster than traditional statistical methods, and therefore are valuable tools for evaluating the effectiveness of a process and ensuring the sustainability of improvements over time.

The control chart: the key tool of SPC

Shewhart developed a relatively simple statistical tool – the control chart – to aid in distinguishing between common and special cause variation. A control chart consists of two parts: (1) a series of measurements plotted in time order, and (2) the control chart "template" which consists of three horizontal lines called the centre line (typically, the mean), the upper control limit (UCL), and the lower control limit (LCL). Examples are shown in Figures 12.1–5. The values of the UCL and LCL are usually calculated from the inherent variation in the data rather than set arbitrarily by the individual making the chart. A firm understanding of the standard distributions used for common cause process variation is therefore essential for the appropriate application of control charts (see later).

To interpret a control chart, data that fall outside the control limits or display abnormal patterns (see later) are indications of special cause variation – that is, it is highly likely that something inherently different in the process led to these data compared with the other data. As long as all values on the graph fall randomly between the upper and lower control limits, however, we assume that we are simply observing common cause variation.

Where to draw the UCL and LCL is important in control chart construction. Shewhart and other SPC experts recommend control limits set at ± 3SD for detecting meaningful changes in process performance while achieving a rational balance between two types of risks. If the limits are set too narrow there is a high risk of a "type I error" – mistakenly inferring special cause variation exists when, in fact, a predictable extreme value is being observed which is expected periodically from common cause variation. This situation is analogous to a false positive indication on a laboratory test. On the other hand, if the limits are set too wide there is a high risk of a "type II error" analogous to a false negative laboratory test.

For example, for the familiar normal distribution, in the long run 99·73% of all plotted data are expected to fall within 3SD of the mean if the process is stable and does not change, with only the remaining 0·27% falling more than 3SD away from the mean. While points that fall outside these limits will occur infrequently due to common cause variation, the type I error probability is so small (0·0027) that we instead conclude that special variation caused these data. Similar logic can be applied to calculate the type I and type II errors for any other statistical distribution.

Although traditional statistical techniques used in the medical literature typically use 2SD as the statistical criterion for making decisions, there are several important reasons why control charts use 3SD. For the normal distribution approximately 95% of the values lie within 2SD of the mean so, even if the process was stable and in control, if control limits are set at 2SD the type I error (false positive) rate for *each* plotted value would be about 5% compared with 0·27% for a 3SD chart. Unlike one time hypothesis tests, however, control charts consist of many points (20–25 is common) with each point contributing to the overall false positive probability. A control chart with 25 points using 3SD control limits has a reasonably acceptable overall false positive probability of $1 - (0{\cdot}9973)^{25} = 6{\cdot}5\%$, whereas using 2SD limits would produce an unacceptably high overall false positive probability of $1 - (0{\cdot}95)^{25} = 27{\cdot}7\%$! The bottom line is that the UCL and LCL are set at 3SD above and below the mean on most common control charts.[5]

In addition to points outside the control limits, we can also look more rigorously at whether data appear randomly distributed between the limits. Statisticians have developed additional tests for this purpose. For example, a common set of tests for special cause variation is:

- one point outside the upper or lower control limits
- two of three successive points more than 2SD from the mean on the same side of the centre line
- four out of five successive points more than 1SD from the mean on the same side of the centre line
- eight successive points on the same side of the centre line;
- six successive points increasing or decreasing (a trend); or
- obvious cyclic behaviour.

In return for a minor increase in false positives, these additional tests greatly increase the power of control charts to detect process improvements and deteriorations. The statistical "trick" here is that we are accumulating information and looking for special cause patterns to form while waiting for the total sample size to increase. This process of accumulating information before declaring statistical significance is powerful, both statistically and psychologically.

A final important point about the construction of control charts concerns the mechanics of calculating the SD. As with traditional statistical methods, many different formulae can be used to calculate the SD depending on the type of control chart used and the particular statistical distribution associated with that chart. In particular, the formula for the SD is *not* the one typically used to calculate the empirical SD as might be found in a computer spreadsheet or taught in a basic statistics class. For example, if we are monitoring the proportion of surgery patients who acquire an infection, the appropriate formulae would use the SD of a binomial distribution (much like that for a conventional hypothesis test of proportions); if monitoring a medication error rate the appropriate formulae would use the SD of a Poisson distribution; and when using normally distributed data the appropriate formulae essentially block on the within sample SD in a manner similar to that used in hypothesis tests of means and variances. Details of calculations for each type of control chart, when to use each chart, and appropriate sample sizes for each type of chart are beyond the scope of this paper but can be found in many standard SPC publications.[5–10]

Examples

The following examples illustrate the basic principles, breadth of application, and versatility of control charts as a data analysis tool.

Flash sterilization rate

The infection control (IC) committee at a 180 bed hospital notices an increase in the infection rate for surgical patients. A nurse on the committee suggests that a possible contributor to this increase is the use of flash sterilisation (FS) in the operating theatres. Traditionally, FS was used only in emergency situations – for example, when an instrument was dropped during surgery – but recently it seems to have become a more routine procedure. Some committee members express the opinion that a new group of orthopaedic surgeons who recently joined the hospital staff might be a contributing factor – that is, special cause variation. This suggestion creates some defensiveness and unease within the committee.

Rather than debating opinions, the committee decides to take a closer look at this hypothesis by analysing some data on the FS rate (number of FS per 100 surgeries) to see how it has varied over time. The committee's analyst prepares a *u* chart (based on the Poisson distribution, Figure 12.1) to determine the hospital's baseline rate and the rate after the arrival of the new surgeons.

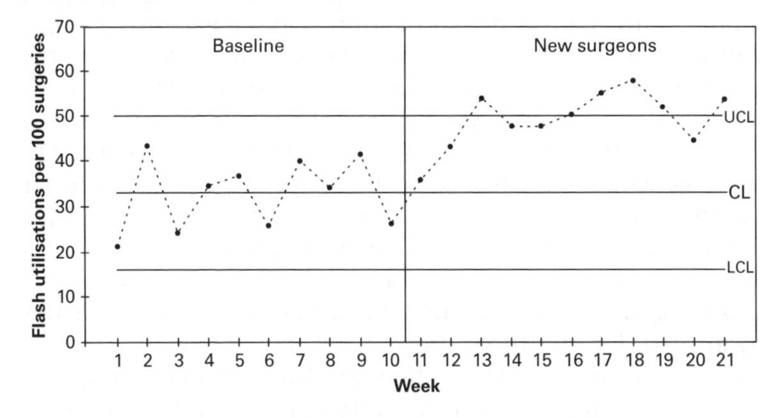

Figure 12.1 Control chart for flash sterilisation rate: baseline compared with period following arrival of new surgical group

During the baseline period the mean FS rate was around 33 per 100 surgeries (the centre line on the baseline control chart) and the process appeared to be in control. However, arrival of the new surgeons indicated an increase (special cause variation) to a mean FS rate of about 50 per 100 surgeries. For example, the third data point (week 13) is beyond the baseline UCL, as are weeks 17, 18, 19, and 21. Additionally, several clusters of two out of three points are more than 2SD beyond the mean, several clusters of four out five points are beyond 1SD, and all of the new points are above the baseline period mean. All these signals are statistical evidence of a significant and sustained shift in process performance. The IC committee can now look further into this matter with confidence that it is not merely an unsupported opinion.

It must be noted that this analysis does not lead to the conclusion that the new surgeons are to *blame* for the increase. Rather, the data simply indicate that it is highly likely that something about the process of handling surgical instruments has fundamentally changed, coincident with the arrival of the new surgeons. Further investigation is warranted.

Laboratory turn around time (TAT)

Several clinicians in the A&E department have been complaining that the turn around time (TAT) for complete blood counts has been "out of control and constantly getting worse". The laboratory manager decides to investigate this assertion with data rather than just opinions. The data are stratified by shift and type of request (urgent versus routine) to ensure that the analysis is conducted by reasonably homogeneous processes. Since TAT data often follow normal distributions, *X-bar* and *S* types of control charts are appropriate here (Figure 12.2). Each day the mean and SD TAT were calculated for three randomly selected orders for complete blood counts. The top chart (*X-bar*) chart shows the mean TAT for the three orders each day, while the bottom chart (*S*) shows the SD for the same three orders; during the day shift the mean time to get results for a routine complete blood count is about 45 minutes with a mean SD of about 21 minutes.

If the clinicians' complaints were true, out of control points and an overall increasing trend would be observed. Instead, it appears that the process is performing consistently and in a state of statistical control. Although this conclusion may not agree with the clinicians' views, common cause variation does not necessarily mean the results are acceptable, but only that the process is stable and predictable. An in control process can therefore be predictably bad.

In this case the process is stable and predictable but not acceptable to the clinicians. Since the process exhibits only common cause variation, it is appropriate to consider improvement strategies to lower the mean TAT and reduce the variation (lower the centre line and bring the control limits closer together). This would produce a new and more acceptable level of performance. The next steps for the team are therefore to test an improvement idea, compare the new process with these baseline measurements, and decide whether the process has improved, stayed the same, or worsened.

Surgical site infections

An interdisciplinary team has been meeting to try to reduce the postoperative surgical site infection (SSI) rate for certain surgical procedures. A *g* type of control chart (based on the geometric distribution) for one type of surgery is shown in Figure 12.3. Instead of aggregating SSIs in order to calculate an

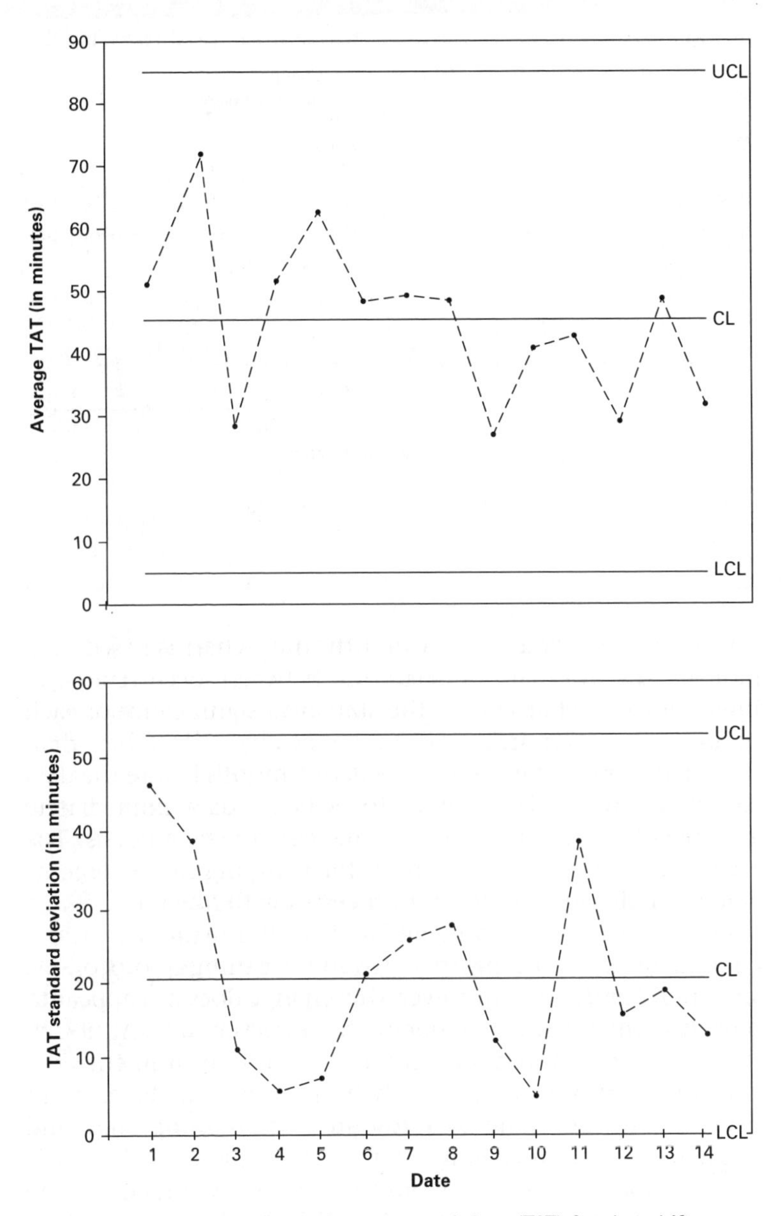

Figure 12.2 Control chart of turn around time (TAT) for day shift routine orders for complete blood counts in the A&E department

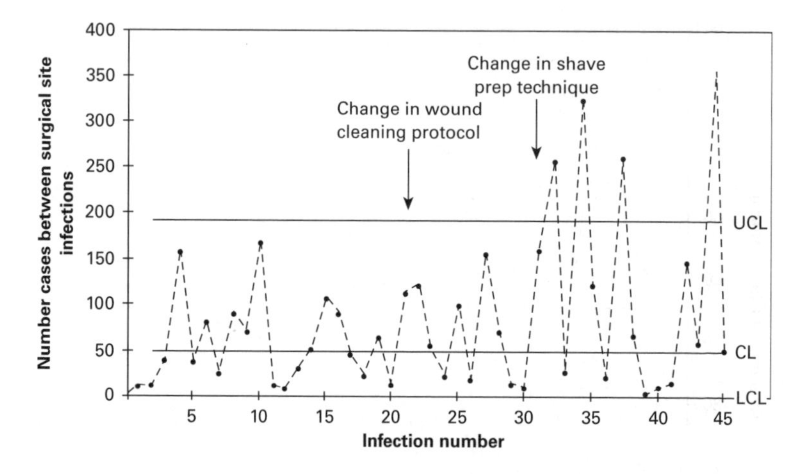

Figure 12.3 Control chart for surgical site infections

infection rate over a week or month, the *g* chart is based on a plot of the number of surgeries between occurrences of infection. This chart allows the statistical significance of each occurrence of an infection to be evaluated[11] rather than having to wait to the end of a week or a month before the data can be analysed. This ability to evaluate data immediately greatly enhances the potential timeliness of the analysis. The *g* chart is also particularly useful for verifying improvements (such as reduced SSIs) and for processes with low rates.

An initial intervention suggested by the team is to test a change in the postoperative wound cleaning protocol. As shown in Figure 12.3, however, this change does not appear to have had any impact on reducing the infection rate. Although this intervention did not result in an improvement, the control chart was useful to help prevent the team from investing further time and resources in training staff and implementing an ineffective change throughout the hospital.

After more brainstorming and review of the literature, the team decided to try experimenting with the shave preparation technique for preparing the surgical site before surgery. Working initially with a few willing surgeons and nurses, they developed a new shave preparation protocol and used it for several months. The control chart in Figure 12.3 indicates that

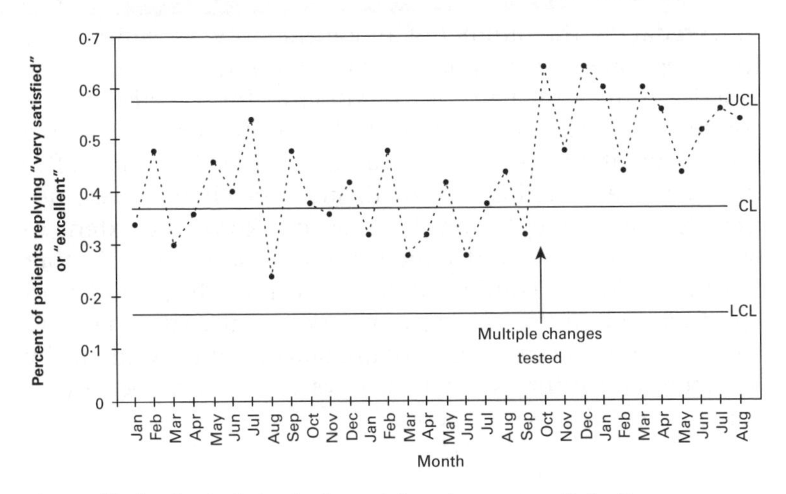

Figure 12.4 Control chart of appointment access satisfaction (percentage of patients very satisfied or higher with delay to see provider)

this change resulted in an improvement with the SSI rate reducing from approximately 2·1% to 0·9%. (For this type of chart the mean SSI rate is the reciprocal of the mean: 1/47 = 2·1% before the change compared with 1/111 = 0·9% after the change.) Note that on this type of chart data plotted above the UCL indicate an improvement, as an increase in the number of surgeries between SSIs equates to a decrease in the SSI rate.

Appointment access satisfaction

A GP practice is working hard on improving appointment access and has decided to track several performance measures each month. A small survey has been developed to gauge patients' satisfaction with several aspects of appointment access (delay, telephone satisfaction, in office waiting times, able to see provider of choice, etc). The percentage of patients who respond "very good" or "excellent" to the question of how satisfied they were with the delay to get an appointment with their primary care provider is plotted on a p control chart (based on the binomial distribution) shown in Figure 12.4.

After exploring ideas that had been successful for other practices, the staff implemented several changes at the same time: reducing the number of appointment types, simplifying the telephone scripts, and offering appointments with the practice nurse in lieu of the doctor for certain minor conditions. As shown in the control chart, there was a notable improvement in appointment access satisfaction soon after these changes were implemented. Since the changes were not tried one at a time, however, we do not know the extent to which each change contributed to the improvement; further testing could be conducted to determine this, similar in approach to traditional screening experiments. This chart can also be used to monitor the sustainability of improvements by detecting any future special cause variation of a decrease in appointment access satisfaction.

Infectious waste monitoring

If several staff were asked to identify the criteria for determining what constitutes infectious waste in a hospital, a wide variety of responses would probably be obtained. Faced with this lack of standardization, most hospitals spend more time and money disposing of infectious waste than is necessary. For example, recent studies in the USA found that less than 6% of a hospital's waste can be considered infectious or hazardous. It has also been estimated that an average size hospital spends the equivalent of a new CAT scanner every year disposing of improperly classified infectious waste such as soft drink cans, paper, milk cartons, and disposable gowns. Armed with this knowledge, a team decides to address this issue.

Since the team had no idea how much infectious waste they produced each day, they first established a baseline. As shown on the left side of Figure 12.5 (an *XmR* chart based on the normal distribution), the mean daily amount of infectious waste during the baseline period was a little over 7 lb (3·2 kg). The process was stable and exhibited only common cause variation, so an intervention improvement strategy is appropriate. If the process is not changed, the amount of infectious waste in future weeks might be expected to vary between 6 lb (2·8 kg) and 8·2 lb (3·7 kg) per day. To reduce the mean amount of infectious waste produced daily, the team

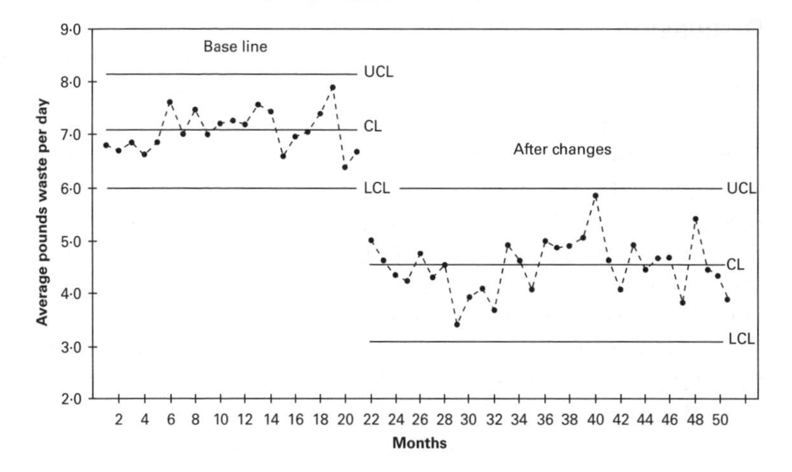

Figure 12.5 Control chart of infectious waste

first established a clear operational definition of infectious waste and then conducted an educational campaign to make everyone more aware of what was and was not infectious waste. They next developed posters, designed tent cards for the cafeteria tables, made announcements at departmental meetings, and assembled displays of inappropriate items found in the infectious waste containers. The results of this educational effort are shown on the right side of Figure 12.5. The process has shifted to a new and more acceptable level of performance. Since the process has clearly changed, new control limits have been calculated for the data after the improvement. The new mean daily production of infectious waste is a little more than 4 lb (1·8 kg) per day.

The control chart provided the team with a useful tool for testing the impact of these efforts. In this case, the shift in the process was very noticeable and in the desired direction. It is interesting, however, that, although the mean amount of waste was reduced, these same improvements inadvertently also caused the day to day variation to increase (note the wider control limits). Not all changes lead to the desired results. A challenge for the team now is to reduce the variation back to at least its original level.

Discussion

These examples illustrate several general points about control charts. Control charts can be used in the daily management of healthcare processes to analyse routinely collected data and reduce "management by opinion", as in the cases of flash sterilisation and laboratory turn around time. Control charts can help policy makers avoid wasted investments in changes that sound good but do not actually deliver, as was the case in the surgical site infection example. That case further illustrated how control charts might be able to detect statistically significant signals from the patterns in the data more quickly than traditional statistical methods. The appointment access satisfaction example illustrated the general application of control charts for conducting rapid screening experiments as an efficient prelude to a more traditional experiment.[12] The infectious waste example illustrated the advantage of control charts for a layperson to see the statistical significance of both the shift in the mean and the change in the variability of the measurement under study.

More generally, these examples illustrate how control charts help teams to decide on the correct improvement strategy – whether to search for special causes (if the process is out of control) or to work on more fundamental process improvements and redesign (if the process is in control). In each example the control charts can also be used as a simple monitoring aid to assure that improvements are sustained over time.

One of the benefits of using control charts is that they do not require as much data as traditional statistical analysis which relies on large aggregated data sets. For example, the *g* chart in Figure 12.3 uses each incident of infection as a data point for decision making, the *X-bar* and *S* charts in Figure 12.2 are based on samples of three randomly selected laboratories per day, and the *u* chart in Figure 12.1 uses rates based on the mean of 80 surgeries per week performed in the hospital. Generally speaking, 20–30 such data points are needed to calculate the UCL and LCL, but after that each new data point can be judged for its statistical significance. The exact number of data points needed to construct a reasonable chart will depend on: (1) the type of chart being used; (2) the manner in which the data have been organized and collected; (3) the distributional characteristics of the data – for example, if it is suspected that the data contain extremes (skewness) it would be wise to collect 25–30 data points before calculating the control limits; and (4) the importance of detecting a process change rapidly (the greater the importance, the larger the sample).

Each of the charts used in the examples presented here is based on a different underlying random distribution model. There are at least a dozen different types of control charts in common use in manufacturing and other industries, with three or four new types being developed each year. The various types differ by the statistic plotted – for example, means, percentages, counts, moving means, cumulative sums, interval between events, etc – and the distribution assumed – for example, normal, binomial, Poisson, geometric, etc. Other control charts have been developed for special purpose applications – for example, naturally cyclic processes, short run processes, start up processes, risk adjustment applications, rare events. All have different formulae for calculating centre lines and control limits.

Regardless of the complexity or underlying statistical theory, however, most control charts have the same visual appearance (a chronological graph of frequent process data with a centre line, UCL, and LCL) and are interpreted in a similar way as discussed above. Moreover, experience in a variety of industries outside health care indicates that individuals with little formal statistical training can use control charts to bring more statistical rigour to their decision making.

Conclusions

Control charts are powerful, user friendly, and statistically rigorous process analysis tools that can be used by quality improvement researchers and practitioners alike. These tools can help managers, process improvement practitioners, and researchers to use objective data and statistical thinking to make appropriate decisions.

Key messages

- Measurement data from healthcare processes display natural variation which can be modelled using a variety of statistical distributions.
- Distinguishing between natural "common cause" variation and significant "special cause" variation is key both to knowing how to proceed with improvement and whether or not a change has resulted in real improvement.
- Statistical process control (SPC) is a branch of statistics comparable in rigour and validity to traditional statistical methods.
- Control charts (tools of SPC) can often yield insights into data more quickly and in a way more understandable to the lay decision maker than traditional statistical methods.

References

1 Berwick DM. Harvesting knowledge from improvement. *JAMA* 1996; **275**:877–8.
2 Campbell D, Stanley J. *Experimental and quasi-experimental designs*. Houghton Mifflin, 1963.
3 Shewhart WA. *The economic control of quality of manufactured product*. New York: Van Nostrand, 1931.
4 Deming WE. *Out of the crisis*. Cambridge, MA: Massachusetts Institute of Technology Center for Advanced Engineering Studies, 1986.
5 Benneyan JC. Statistical quality control methods in infection control and epidemiology. Part 2: Chart use, statistical properties, and research issues. *Infect Control Hosp Epidemiol* 1998;**19**:265–83.
6 Grant EL, Leavenworth RS. *Statistical quality control*. 6th ed. New York: McGraw-Hill, 1988.
7 Montgomery DC. *Introduction to statistical quality control*. 2nd ed. New York: Wiley, 1991.
8 Carey RG, Lloyd RC. *Measuring quality improvement in healthcare: a guide to statistical process control applications*. Milwaukee, WI: American Society for Quality, Quality Press, 2001.
9 Plsek P. Tutorial: introduction to control charts. *Qual Manage Health Care* 1992;**1**:65–73.
10 Benneyan JC. Use and interpretation of statistical quality control charts. *Int J Qual Health Care* 1998;**10**:69–73.
11 Benneyan JC. Number-between g-type statistical control charts for monitoring adverse events. *Health Care Manage Sci* 2001;**4**:305–18.
12 Campbell M, Fitzpatrick R, Haines A, *et al*. Framework for design and evaluation of complex interventions to improve health. *BMJ* 2000; **321**:694–6.

13: Value for money of changing healthcare services? Economic evaluation of quality improvement

JOHAN L SEVERENS

There are many instances of perceived or real inefficiencies in health service delivery. Both healthcare providers and policy makers need to know the impact and cost of applying strategies to change the behaviour of individuals or organisations. Quality improvement or implementation research is a branch of health service research concerned with evaluating the methods of behavioural change. Addressing inefficiencies in healthcare services raises a series of issues, beginning with how inefficiency itself should be defined and described. In this paper basic concepts of cost analysis and economic evaluations are explained and a model for working through the economic issues of quality improvement is discussed. This model combines the costs and benefits of corrected inefficiency with the costs and degree of behavioural change achieved by a quality improvement method in the policy maker's locality. It shows why it may not always be cost effective for policy makers to address suboptimal behaviour. Both the interpretation of quality improvement research findings and their local application need careful consideration. The limited availability of applicable quality improvement research may make it difficult currently to provide robust advice on the value for money of many behavioural quality improvement strategies.

There are a number of formal definitions of "inefficiency", but broadly we can think of it as a wasteful use of resources for no (or very little) benefit or a failure to use resources on clearly beneficial activities. Inefficiency may arise because of apparently inappropriate, irrational, or misinformed decisions by individuals (carers, patients, or clinicians) or organisations. The impact of non-compliance on healthcare efficiency is determined by its effects on both outcome and costs.[1] Quality improvement and implementation methods seek to change the behaviour of individuals or organisations in response to inefficiencies. Behavioural change comes at a certain cost and achieves a certain level of change. It is never costless – for example, the pharmaceutical industry markets and supports its products to influence uptake and these costs are offset against increased profit. From a social perspective, we need to assess health gains which we commonly think of in physical rather than monetary terms. A more complex framework than simple net profit is therefore needed. The economics of quality improvement provide a way of thinking about inefficiency and identify, for policy makers and practitioners, the best use of scarce resources to achieve quality improvement goals. There are many instances of apparent inefficiencies and variation in our healthcare systems, resulting in considerable interest from policy makers about the scope for using quality improvement and change management methods. Examples include important research findings that do not translate consistently into practice, older but cost effective treatments that fall out of fashion, or equivocal but well marketed products that achieve considerable uptake.[2,3,4] This paper describes an introduction to economic evaluations and presents models and examples of economic evaluations of quality improvement and implementation strategies in health care.

Basics of economic evaluation of healthcare interventions

Economic evaluations are a specific form of evaluation research which focus on making the relationship explicit between the amount of benefit achieved and the required investment related to a healthcare intervention. Before an evaluation can be considered a complete and valuable economic evaluation, two criteria must be met. First, there needs to be a problem of choice. In quality improvement research this problem of choice consists of a comparison of different quality improvement strategies or the comparison of such a strategy and "doing nothing" or "usual health care". Second, in economic evaluations an explicit relationship is made between the efforts (use of people and resources), on the one hand, and the related consequences or actual outcomes on the other. The use of people and resources is usually expressed in monetary units (euros, dollars) so that they can be considered expenses. Relating costs to outcome results in the efficiency or relative cost effectiveness of a quality improvement strategy which can be expressed as a cost effectiveness ratio.[5] An example is shown in Box 13.1.

Box 13.1 Example: A randomised study of three training/support strategies for physicians to use when screening and intervening in cases of alcohol abuse[5]

The three training/support strategies were intended to motivate physicians to introduce screening and a brief intervention targeted towards alcohol abuse. The strategies concerned were (1) distribution of guidelines, (2) distribution of guidelines plus training, and (3) distribution of guidelines plus training and telephone support. Strategy 3 was the most cost effective in terms of cost per patient screened and cost per patient on whom an intervention had been performed. The cost effectiveness for each strategy was determined separately. Costs per patient screened were: trained and supported GPs (£1·05); trained GPs (£1·08); and controls (£1·47). Costs per patient in whom an intervention had been performed were: trained and supported GPs (£5·43); trained GPs (£6·02); and controls (£8·19). The cost effectiveness reported therefore concerned the relative cost effectiveness compared with doing nothing, an alternative which was not included in the study.

Incremental analysis of these figures indicated that the relative cost effectiveness of distribution of the guidelines plus training versus guideline distribution only is more positive than the relative cost effectiveness of distribution of the guidelines plus training and telephone support versus guideline distribution only. The relative cost effectiveness of the most intensive form of implementation (distribution of guidelines plus training and telephone support) compared with distribution of guidelines plus training turned out to be less preferable.

Cost analysis

The execution of cost analyses is the main part of each economic evaluation of quality improvement strategies. Within a cost analysis a distinction is made between fixed and variable costs. Fixed costs are costs that show no link to the scale of the actual use of the specific (healthcare) provision. For example, if consensus meetings are organised to formulate a clinical guideline, the costs will remain the same whether the guideline is later used by one or 100 primary care physicians/ general practitioners (GPs) or whether it is applicable to 100 or 1000 patients. Attribution of fixed costs to an individual caregiver or an individual patient occurs on the basis of a division. If we assume the fixed costs to amount to €10 000 for the consensus meetings and there are 10 physicians with 10 relevant patients each, the fixed costs for that guideline are €1000 per healthcare provider and €100 per patient.

On the one hand, the variable costs of a quality improvement strategy are dependent on the intensity. For example, extra education that lasts more than one day is more expensive than extra education that lasts only a few hours. On the other hand, the variable costs are related to the degree to which the guideline or change proposal is followed. Let us assume that a guideline advises that patients with a high risk for cardiovascular disease should be recalled on a regular basis for check ups to measure blood pressure. In this case, the number of patients affected by the guideline determines the costs involved. If the number of patients is zero, then the number of clinical actions based on the guidelines is zero, and thus there are zero costs. Variable costs will therefore always have to be measured empirically because they cannot be calculated through a simple division per measuring unit (practice, primary care physician, or patient), as can be done with fixed costs.

Different types of costs

In the economic evaluation of quality improvement interventions, costs can be subdivided into different phases of the quality improvement process.[6] Firstly, there are costs related to the task of collecting evidence to identify best practices or to the task of developing new or optimal care procedures. Patient related research can be performed, for example, so that best care procedures can be defined and consensus meetings can be organised in order to collect the opinions of experts in the specific area of attention. Basically, these *developmental costs* (fixed costs) should be part of a cost analysis regarding quality improvement strategies in case a change and improvement intervention is not available and has to be developed or adjusted.

Secondly, there are costs associated with *organising a specific quality improvement or change intervention*. For example, when implementing a clinical guideline that uses outreach visitors who are to visit primary care physicians, their training would be desirable. Such costs are basically one-time costs and can therefore be considered fixed costs, unless the intervention used after the experience that is gained is subject to change. In that case, the efforts associated with a revision of the strategy must be considered execution costs.

On the other hand, the costs of the actual *execution of the quality improvement strategy* (such as sending out guidelines or outreach visitors who spend time visiting GP practices) are not relevant until the moment the strategy is executed.[7] Such costs can be considered fixed or variable, depending on the amount of detail included in the cost study. If researchers perform a general cost analysis and use a fixed cost approach, it will be sufficient to know the total scale of the outreach visitor formation. Consequently, a division calculation can be made based on the number of GPs or patients reached (depending on the level of cost effectiveness measuring which is discussed later). It is then, however, not possible to determine cost variation per GP or patient. If the researchers want to determine such a variation to obtain more detail, each outreach visitor will have to record the time spent per visit. With that information, the variable costs can be determined per visit, per practice, per physician, and possibly even per patient. Obviously, a combination of the fixed and variable costs approximation is possible: the visitors' time that is not directly related to a physician's clinical work (such as work meetings and reading of literature) are considered fixed (overhead) costs and attributed to each specific visitor by using a division calculation. The time that is directly related to the visit of a specific practice is expressed in minutes and converted into monetary units. Examples are shown in Boxes 13.2 and 13.3.

Box 13.2 Example: Costs and cost reductions of a quality strategy to improve test ordering in general practice[6]

This multicentre randomised controlled trial compared the costs and cost reductions of an innovative strategy aimed at improving the test ordering routines of GPs with a traditional strategy. It included 27 local GP groups in the Netherlands with diagnostic centres and comprised a total of 194 GPs. The test ordering strategy was systematically developed and combined feedback, guideline dissemination, and quality improvement sessions in small groups. In 13 experimental local groups, GPs discussed their feedback report at regular quality meetings, related them to guidelines, and made plans for change. In 14 control groups only feedback was provided. The main outcome measures were costs, which were divided into running costs (costs of the feedback reports), development costs (activities for the continuation of the project – administration, organisation, development and updating of concise guideline information), and research costs (activities for the scientific development of the feedback system). In addition, costs (reductions) of the laboratory tests and all tests per GP and per 6 months were determined by assessing the difference between the follow up period and the baseline period in the costs of tests ordered; this difference was compared between the two arms.

When only running costs were included, the total strategy was found to cost €93 per GP per 6 months compared with €17 per GP per 6 months in the feedback arm. The GPs in the total strategy arm achieved a mean reduction in the costs of tests of €301 per GP per 6 months compared with €161 per GP per 6 months in the feedback arm. On the basis of this cost analysis, the authors recommended the implementation of the quality strategy on a larger scale.

This study clearly shows that not only developmental and execution costs are relevant in economic evaluation, but also the costs related to the change in healthcare provision. Of course, limiting the analysis of the costs of healthcare provision to diagnostic activities and not including the costs of therapeutic actions is based on the assumption that this would increase the positive cost difference found.

Box 13.3 Example: Process evaluation of a multifaceted intervention to improve cardiovascular disease prevention in general practice[7]

The Dutch CARPE study was a randomised controlled before and after study which evaluated quality improvement resulting from the use of trained consultants for patients with cardiovascular risk indicators or cardiovascular disease in 60 experimental and 60 control GP

(Continued)

Box 13.3 *(Continued)*

practices. Before and after the quality improvement strategy was applied, measurements were taken of the organisational characteristics (teamwork, special office hours, administrative and patient follow up systems), the healthcare process (working according to GP standards), and clinical parameters (blood pressure, etc). The implementation strategy consisted of regular visits by trained consultants to the experimental practices during an 18 month period. The consultants' task was to encourage the active use of seven national primary care physician/medical guidelines (hypertension, cholesterol, diabetes mellitus II, peripheral arteriosclerosis, angina pectoris, heart failure, and cerebrovascular accident or TIA).

The cost of this implementation strategy was compared with the cost of no active implementation strategy over an 18 month period from the healthcare perspective. The cost analysis was limited to the execution of the implementation strategy, so possible changes in the healthcare process (such as longer consultations) were not taken into consideration. It was therefore not necessary to perform cost research in the control practices since the cost of no implementation strategy would equal zero by definition.

During the study the costs for each visit to the GP practices were prospectively recorded by the consultant. This included the number of visits by the consultant to each practice; the preparation, travel, and consultation time per visit; the preparation and execution time spent by the GP(s) and practice assistant(s) during each consultant visit; and the number of miles the consultant had to travel. The recorded activities were compared with the actual cost prices. Data were collected on 934 consultation visits to 62 GP practices. Even though the protocol required a fixed number of consultation visits per practice, the actual number of visits per practice ranged from 3 to 17 (mean 14·8). Partly because of this, the costs per practice varied. It also turned out that the number of primary care physicians and assistants who actively participated in the implementation strategy by preparing and attending consultation visits varied for each practice from one to four primary care physicians and zero to five assistants per practice. In particular, the costs of time investment of the primary care physicians largely determined the variation in costs of the quality improvement strategy.

The above mentioned cost categories are the cost per practice or caregiver of a quality improvement strategy (as reflected by Δc_i in the model described by Mason et al[8]). In addition, costs are sometimes associated with a *change in healthcare provision* as a result of application of a quality improvement strategy. As a result of the application of a clinical guideline, for instance, physicians may be able to see patients more frequently or consultations may last longer because of more elaborate physical examinations. Benefits may include the ability to perform more diagnostic tests and the possibility of a quicker referral of a patient to the specialist. This also includes a change in the way a patient makes use of medical care, which can be partly attributed to effects on health. Non-medical costs, such as patients' cost for time and travel and costs resulting from absence from work, can also be analysed on this level. These changes in healthcare provision costs are always considered variable costs. In essence, they are part of the cost of care (as reflected by Δc_t in the model of Mason et al[8]).

Different types of economic evaluations

The process or patient outcome (consequences, benefits) of alternative strategies studied in quality improvement projects are sometimes similar, in which case a cost minimisation analysis is useful (Box 13.4).[9] However, in most quality improvement strategies process or patient outcomes are also relevant, in addition to costs, and a full economic evaluation should be performed. The expression of the ratio of costs versus consequences into one unit (the cost effectiveness ratio) is often neglected when evaluating quality improvement strategies. Such studies can be called "cost consequence analyses" and simply give an overview of the costs and consequences without connecting them into one single unit. They are then presented to policy makers who have to make a decision about the choice of intervention based on a list of pros and cons without indicating a value or preference.[10] McIntosh et al[11] introduced the so called "balance sheet approach" in which positive and negative consequences are simply stated in a table. Although useful, these methods do not give a clear insight into the question of efficiency, which is the aim of other types of economic evaluation.

Box 13.4 Example: Individual feedback to physicians about diagnostic test requests[9]

In this study the influence of individual feedback on physicians' requests for diagnostic tests was examined. Based on an extensive retrospective study, it was shown that the individual feedback led to

(Continued)

Box 13.4 ***(Continued)***

a significant reduction in costs. In order to estimate the relative impact of the implementation strategy, data were used from a comparable laboratory in another part of The Netherlands. The researchers concluded that, based on both retrospective comparison and on the comparison with data from the other laboratory, routine individual feedback can be considered economically valuable. Data on patient outcomes were not available. Possible undesired side effects of the decline in diagnostic test requests were described on the basis of the number of hospital referrals in which no unexpected changes had been observed. Since no explicit connection was made between costs and outcomes, this study can be defined as a cost minimisation analysis. Although not stated, it was implied that cheaper health care would not equal worse health care.

Cost effectiveness analyses express effects in natural quantitative parameters which can be process parameters[12] as well as patient outcome measures. In quality improvement research this may include, among others, the number of practices reached by the quality improvement strategy (for example, mailing of guidelines); the number of practices, departments, or professionals working in accordance with a specific clinical guideline or care pathway; the number of patients receiving treatment in accordance with such a guideline; the health condition of the patients concerned; and their satisfaction with the health care provided. An example of cost effectiveness analysis in thrombosis is shown in Box 13.5.

Box 13.5 Example: Cost effectiveness of audit in thrombosis[12]

A study that examined the cost effectiveness of audit in improving the care of patients suspected of having an acute myocardial infarction provides an example of the problems concerning process parameters versus patient outcomes as cost effectiveness parameters. This study examined the cost of each additional patient treated for thrombosis. Instead of patient outcomes, a process parameter was used which resulted in an estimate of £101–395 per additional patient treated. The authors rightly based their choice for such an outcome measure on the fact that there is overwhelming evidence that the clinical actions encouraged are effective and pragmatic. This legitimised the assumption that the increase in thrombosis treatment would lead to better patient outcome, although this was not explicitly analysed.

In cost utility analysis the physical health of the patient as an outcome measure is central. In these analyses the patient's eventual physical health is rated through the use of a utility. This physical health rating is indicated by a number between 0 and 1, where 1 equals perfect health and 0 the worst imaginable condition (death). Utilities can be used as the basis for the calculation of so called quality adjusted life years (QALYs), a measure that uses societal rating of a patient's health and relates it to life span (Box 13.6). In general, cost utility analyses require a lot of work because patients are required to fill out extensive questionnaires. This method of analysis is applied frequently in clinical evaluation studies but only occasionally in quality improvement or implementation research.[13]

Box 13.6 Example: Randomised controlled economic evaluation of asthma self-management in primary health care[13]

In this randomised controlled economic evaluation, guided self-management of asthma was compared with usual asthma care according to guidelines for Dutch family physicians. Nineteen family practices were randomised and 193 adults with stable asthma (98 self-management, 95 usual care) were included and monitored for 2 years. Patient specific cost data were collected, preference based utilities were assessed, and incremental cost per quality adjusted life year (QALY) and incremental cost per successfully treated week gained was calculated. Self-management patients gained 0·039 QALY and experienced 81 successfully treated weeks during the 2 year period; the corresponding figures for usual care were 0·024 QALY and 75 weeks. Total costs were 1084 euros for self-management and 1097 euros for usual care. Self-management patients consumed 1680 puffs of budesonide compared with 1897 by those in the usual care group. When all costs were included, self-management was cost effective on all outcomes. It was concluded that guided self-management is a safe and efficient alternative approach compared with the asthma treatment usually provided in Dutch primary care.

Finally, cost benefit analyses are distinguished from other types of economic evaluations because they measure, not only the costs, but also the consequences in financial terms. For example, a patient's survival or quality of life is expressed in guilders or dollars. There are many issues involved in this and therefore cost benefit analyses are seldom used in health care. The term "cost benefit" is often used incorrectly because financial savings that are characterised as benefits are, in fact, lower costs.

The efficiency or cost effectiveness of a quality improvement strategy expresses how the costs relate to the results obtained. These can then be formulated as the intervention costs per optimally treated patient (process parameters as outcome unit) or as change or implementation costs plus treatment costs per successfully treated patient (outcome parameter as outcome unit). By comparing the effects and costs of alternative quality improvement strategies with each other, the incremental cost effectiveness ratio can be determined. Based on the comparable alternative in the study, the average amount of investment needed when applying the experimental alternative can be determined.

Model for assessing the overall policy impact of a quality improvement method

From the above description of the different types of economic evaluations it is clear that the ultimate goal of health economists is to express efficiency of a quality improvement strategy in terms of patient outcome. However, to date, this goal has seldom been attained in economic research on quality improvement. An important step forward to overcome this has been made by Mason and colleagues[8] who have developed a more advanced approach to the economic evaluation of quality improvement strategies. Pursuing a policy to change suboptimal patterns of care combines quality improvement cost effectiveness (net cost and magnitude of impact upon behaviour when using a quality improvement strategy) with treatment cost effectiveness (incremental costs and benefits of more optimal behaviour). An example of the estimation of overall policy costs and benefits is shown in the following equation:

Policy cost-effectiveness:

$$\Delta CE_p = \frac{1}{d.n_p.p_d.\Delta b_t} . \Delta CE_i + \Delta CE_t = L_{CE} + \Delta CE_t$$

where Δb_t, Δc_t and ΔCE_t are the net health gain, cost of care and treatment cost effectiveness per patient ($\Delta c_t / \Delta b_t$); Δc_i,

Δb_i and ΔCE_i are the net cost, proportion of patient care changed, and quality improvement cost effectiveness per practice ($\Delta c_i / \Delta b_i$); d is the duration of effect of the quality improvement method; n_p and p_d are the average practice size and population prevalence of the condition targeted; and L_{CE} is the loading factor on treatment cost effectiveness.

This equation shows the case when a change in health care is valued as a cost effectiveness ratio (cost per year of life gained) and the performance marker is the simple proportion of patients receiving appropriate care. This model was used, for example, to analyse data in a study of the apparent underutilisation of ACE inhibitors for heart failure in primary care.[14,15] This so called EBOR trial examined the effectiveness of outreach visits to primary care by community pharmacists using recommendations derived from evidence based clinical practice guidelines. The numbers from the EBOR trial can be put into the equation as follows[8]:

$$\Delta CE_t = \frac{690}{0{\cdot}48} = £1440 \text{ per Life Year}$$

$$\Delta CE_i = \frac{405}{0{\cdot}05} = £7790 \text{ per percent behavioural change}$$

$$\begin{aligned}\Delta CE_p &= \frac{1}{1 \times 5690 \times 0{\cdot}009 \times 0{\cdot}48} \times 7790 + 1440 \\ &= 300 + 1440 = £1740 \text{ per Life Year}\end{aligned}$$

Investing resources to change clinician behaviour imposes an addition (or loading) on treatment cost effectiveness. The loading is small (£300/life year gained) in the example and does not substantially diminish the attractiveness of the intervention to policy makers. Policy cost effectiveness is most likely to remain attractive in those treatments that are highly cost effective, and most likely to become unattractive when the cost effectiveness of treatment is borderline. A potentially complex interplay of factors determines whether quality improvement by a particular method is worthwhile. Cheaper methods achieving greater levels of change reduce the loading effect. Similarly, larger health gains per patient, higher prevalence of disease, larger practice size, or longer duration of behavioural change all reduce the loading, all other things being equal. Where the loading is small, treatment and policy cost effectiveness are very similar. Where the loading is large, further use of a cost effective treatment may not be worthwhile encouraging as a policy goal using available behavioural change methods.

Discussion

Compared with simple treatment interventions, economic evaluations regarding quality improvement strategies are few. Because it is hardly ever possible to have one empirical study that gathers all the data needed to study cost effectiveness of a quality improvement strategy, the model described by Mason et al[8] may provide the solution. In this model a distinction is made between treatment cost effectiveness (the net costs and benefits of a treatment when provided) and policy cost effectiveness (which combines treatment cost effectiveness with the cost and magnitude of change achieved by a quality improvement method). The example presented illustrates the case of a level of efficiency determined by a simple proportion – that is, the percentage of patients receiving an ACE inhibitor. In other instances it may be necessary to consider a mean level of exposure or a combination of dose and proportion. The key is to have robust linkage with (change in) an efficiency measure and treatment costs and health benefit. In addition, with the knowledge of the relative cost effectiveness of following a guideline compared with not following it, it is possible to determine the maximum financial resources that can be used neutrally to encourage the use of a guideline.[16]

A number of assumptions are often implicit when planning quality improvement. Commonly, local patients are assumed to be typical of those enrolled in trials and are treated in the same way. The findings of quality improvement studies are assumed to be transferable to different settings and possibly also to different evidence based messages and diseases. Costs of treatment and quality improvement will vary with the setting, hence the value of studies that report units of component resources disaggregated from their unit costs. The local cost of quality improvement needs to reflect local resource utilisation patterns and prices. The magnitude of behavioural change is unlikely to remain constant over time,[17] and a decision needs to be taken as to whether quality improvement is a "one off" or whether periodic reimplementation needs to be costed.

Prerequisites for worthwhile behavioural change are evidence of local suboptimal care and a locally deliverable cost effective alternative, but the local demography and characteristics of the audience to be targeted may also be important. Failure to understand these facets beforehand risks investment in quality improvement for a poor return. To understand how any piece of quality improvement research may be generalisable to a different context, it is necessary to consider its setting, its message, the method used, facilitators, barriers, and motivations both of those receiving the intervention and those designing it. A trial of educational outreach by community pharmacists to improve general practice prescribing of non-steroidal anti-inflammatory drugs failed to show a significant impact because participating practices already exhibited good baseline prescribing.[18] It is important to address actual rather than perceived problems.

Given their limitations, findings of current quality improvement studies should be applied cautiously. It would be ideal for any condition with known prevalence and method of behavioural change to estimate loading adjustments for treatment cost effectiveness and thus determine the best quality improvement method to meet policy aims. Better research into economic aspects of quality improvement methods is needed to achieve this goal.

Key messages

- Economic evaluations of quality improvement strategies are based on the comparison of alternative methods of introducing desirable changes (or doing nothing) in health care. When performing a complete economic evaluation, the costs incurred by people and resources are related to the (health) outcomes obtained.
- In contrast to economic evaluations of medical interventions, both process and patient outcomes can be used as cost effectiveness measures in economic evaluations of quality improvement strategies.
- Economic evaluation research of quality improvement strategies is most beneficial if the cost effectiveness of the desired professional behaviours or healthcare processes are known and found to be acceptable.
- To determine the cost effectiveness of a quality improvement strategy, the costs and benefits of corrected inefficiency can be combined with the costs and degree of behavioural change in the policy maker's locality.

Acknowledgements

The author is grateful to Professor James Mason, Centre for Health Services Research, University of Newcastle upon Tyne, UK who supported this work substantially, especially by providing the example of the model for assessing the overall policy impact of a quality improvement method, and Dr Michel Wensing, Centre for Quality of Care Research, University Medical Centre Nijmegen, The Netherlands who commented and made suggestions on a previous draft of the paper.

References

1 Cleemput I, Kesteloot K. Economic implications of non-compliance in health care. *Lancet* 2002;**359**:2129–30.
2 Freemantle N, Harvey E, Grimshaw J, Oxman AD. The effectiveness of printed educational materials in changing the behaviour of health care professionals. In: Freemantle N, Bero L, Grilli R, *et al*, eds. *Effective Professional Practice Module of the Cochrane Database of Systematic Reviews. Cochrane Library*, Issue 3. Oxford: Update Software, 1996.
3 Antman E, Lau J, Kupelnick B, *et al.* A comparison of results of meta-analyses of randomized control trials and recommendations of clinical experts. *JAMA* 1992;**268**:240–8.
4 Freemantle N, Mason JM. Is all publicity good publicity? A review of the Prozac years. *PharmacoEconomics* 2000;**17**:319–24.
5 Kaner EFS, Lock CA, McAvoy BR, *et al.* An RCT of three training and support strategies to encourage implementation of screening and brief alcohol intervention by general practitioners. *Br J Gen Pract* 1999;**49**:699–703.
6 Verstappen WHJM, Merode GG van, Grimshaw GM, *et al.* Costs and cost reductions of a quality strategy to improve test ordering in general practice. 2003 (unpublished).
7 Lobo CM, Euser L, Kamp J, *et al.* Process evaluation of a multifaceted intervention to improve cardiovascular disease prevention in general practice. *Eur J Gen Pract* 2003 (in press).
8 Mason J, Freemantle N, Nazareth I, *et al.* When is it cost-effective to change the behaviour of health professionals? *JAMA* 2001;**286**:2988–92.
9 Winkens RAG, Ament A, Pop P. Routine individual feedback on requests for diagnostic tests: an economic evaluation. *Med Decis Making* 1996;**16**: 309–14.
10 Mauskopf JA, Paul JE, Grant DM, *et al.* The role of cost-consequence analysis in health care decision making. *PharmacoEconomics* 1998;**13**: 277–88.
11 McIntosh E, Donaldson C, Ryan M. Recent advances in the methods of cost-benefit analysis in health care. *PharmacoEconomics* 1999;**15**:357–67.
12 Robinson MB, Thompson E, Black NA. Why is the evaluation of the cost-effectiveness of audit so difficult? The example of thrombolysis for suspected acute myocardial infarction. *Qual Health Care* 1998;**7**:19–26.
13 Schermer TR, Thoonen BP, van de Boom G, *et al.* Randomized controlled economic evaluation of asthma self-management in primary health care. *Am J Respir Crit Care Med* 2002;**166**:1062–72.

14 Freemantle N, Eccles M, Wood J, *et al.* A randomised trial of evidence-based outreach (EBOR): rationale and design. *Controlled Clinical Trials* 1999;**20**: 479–92.
15 Freemantle N, Nazareth I, Eccles M, *et al.* A randomised trial of the effect of educational outreach by community pharmacists on prescribing in primary care. *Br J Gen Pract* 2002;**52**:290–5.
16 Sculpher M. Evaluating the cost-effectiveness of interventions designed to increase the utilization of evidence-based guidelines. *Fam Pract* 2000;**17**(Suppl 1):S26–31.
17 Durieux P, Nizard R, Ravaud P, *et al.* A clinical decision support system for prevention of venous thromboembolism: effect on physician behavior. *JAMA* 2000;**283**:2816–21.
18 Watson MJ, Gunnell D, Peters TJ, *et al.* Guidelines and educational outreach visits from community pharmacists to improve prescribing in general practice: a randomised controlled trial. *J Health Serv Res Policy* 2001;**6**:207–13.

Index

Page numbers in **bold** type refer to figures, those in *italics* refer to tables or boxed material